RESUME OF A MALE NURSE

RESUME OF A MALE NURSE

Curtis William Price - L.V.N.

ISBN: 1506164986
ISBN 13: 9781506164984
Library of Congress Control Number: 2015900569
CreateSpace Independent Publishing Platform
North Charleston, South Carolina

Introduction

Never had I set out to become a nurse. Not even a little. It was a decision that came about after becoming the only person to receive my commercial driver's license while working for one of the largest movie-production-equipment-rental warehouses in Hollywood, California.

Why is it that there are some people who are only happy, or at least content, with themselves when others fail at anything they endeavor to achieve? In my opinion they live in an illusion. They need to feel superior, and with the failures of others, they grow stronger in that illusion. If one should succeed, this illusion dissolves equally; that is to say, they lose power. It is the "master and student syndrome." A master is no longer a master when the student achieves anything greater than the master has achieved. Then comes loss with achieving for the achiever. Because no one, master or so-called friend, wishes to keep company with a constant reminder of one's complacency or outright lack of ambition and self-esteem. But in all fairness there are some who sincerely support others. Unfortunately, I have crossed paths with the latter less frequently.

Is life a competition? I believe it is. But for me the competition is only with myself.

I've done the "keeping up with the Joneses." A dead-end street, really, as whatever "it" is will never be enough. I've done the whole waking up, and with the feeling of opening the starting gate, I rush and rush and rush again, and, again, I find I rush to where no one waits. I speak of anxiety, a tangible fear of running out of time. I feel every waking moment should be dedicated to improving myself in the hope of bettering my life and my family's. So I think, and I learn. I move forward because I'm here.

1

Opportunity Knocks

A routine day. A routine workweek. Pulling lights and cables for feature movies, commercials, and videos from the dusty, wooden racks within the movie production equipment-rental warehouse. Great exercise, long days, modest pay on this end. Always keeping my ears and eyes open for opportunities to advance in the entertainment industry. This warehouse encapsulated 90 percent of the equipment needed to make anything celluloid (film).

Opportunity came when all the warehouse men were asked by the head administrative supervisor, Matt, over the intercom, "Who wants to get your commercial driver's license? We need our own Class A drivers for production."

All hands went in the air, including mine. We were told we could come in and punch the clock and get paid for learning, utilize the company commercial vehicles to drive and practice on. Part of my philosophy has been, "If you're not learning, you're not living." That, and if I didn't endeavor in any other occupation, I'd know all too well the answer if someone asked me, "Where do you see yourself in ten years?" My answer could only be the aforementioned dusty racks or getting run over by a bus, neither of which I hoped would happen.

At night I studied the Class A requirements from the Department of Motor Vehicle's commercial driver's handbook. After a few weeks and much questioning from coworkers as to how my education was going, I went to the DMV and failed. They had no gray area when obtaining this license. I was asked about the "slack adjuster," a device used to adjust brakes on commercial vehicles, and I drew a blank. Miss one thing and fail. While demonstrating the driving skills part of the test, should you hit one cone, you fail. I had to wait two weeks before my second attempt.

I drove back after my first try and walked a gauntlet of almost thirty men.

As I walked into the warehouse, I heard, "Knight is back," echoing throughout the warehouse. Matt walked out of the administrative office of carpet and air conditioning into the warehouse of concrete and wooden racks with a half smile of hope on his face.

"Well?" he asked.

"I failed," I replied.

This declaration left my mouth dry. My disappointment in myself angered me.

If it can be read, it can be passed, I thought, clenching my teeth.

Among my audience of thirty men was a man on the grip-equipment side of the warehouse (the warehouse was split into two sides, electrical and grip). "Grips," in movie production, are the people who use light diffusions, colors, and so forth. Stan was about my age, twenty-seven, short in stature and pear shaped. His hair was white and receding. He carried an air of self-importance and was opinionated, with an answer for everything. I believed he had a lack of confidence and that he kept up this delusion of self-glorification (or, at best, his status of "master" in his own mind) so he could feel superior.

Stan said, "I know a lot of people that tried for that license. It's hard, and not many get it. Don't let it get you down."

"Oh, I won't. I'll get it!" I retorted.

His condescending words made me feel that he said this more for himself. To make him feel it was OK not to have tried himself and to have possibly dodged that bullet of humiliation that accompanies failure, and to encourage me to accept defeat and let it go.

The two weeks passed. I had studied every night and drove every day.

I went through the pretest inspection and driving test with the ease of scrambling an egg. The instructor this time was a woman, her appearance as vague now as the day I tested. I focused more on my priorities and gave little room for distractions. I was sitting in the driver's seat of the truck, parked in the DMV parking lot. The instructor sat looking over her paper work. I glanced over without turning my head.

She began, "I would have preferred you spent a little more time on the electrical connections between the tractor and trailer, but all in all, it was an easy pass." She gave me a polite smile as she handed me my results.

Looking at the paper, I saw that all check marks under their specific category of the test were marked "Outstanding" with one exception of a single check in the "Good" category, for electrical connections.

I believe she felt she had to show some deviation from a perfect score. I didn't say anything; I knew it was a perfect score. But I wondered why. Had there never been a perfect score? Or was it her "master" status that she felt I needed to remain below? I drove out of the DMV, grinning and elated, but feeling slightly robbed.

I drove south down the I-5 freeway back to the warehouse. Needless to say, it was well-known that I went to the DMV for my second attempt.

An encore of two weeks earlier played out, this time with a happier ending. The guys came out with their own level of expectations of my success, as did Stan from the grip-equipment side. I was calm and meandered in with a matter-of-fact attitude. Matt again came into the warehouse, the question obvious on his face.

"I got it, Matt," I stated.

A smile replaced his expression of anticipation.

"Great!," he replied.

Then I heard a distinct voice over the hoopla of congratulations.

"I want to see it!" Stan exclaimed.

Almost a dead silence now as all heads turned from me to Stan. He stood in an almost defiant manner. No smile, just a rigid posture with his hands straight down his sides. Slowly, all heads turned their attention back to me. I reached into my back pocket calmly and pulled out my wallet. I opened it and pulled the temporary license out that came via a white slip showing my new classification as a "commercial driver" along with all the endorsements that applied: doubles, triples, tanker, and hazardous materials. I figured, why wait, so I got all the endorsements that went with the category of a Class A license. I lifted my hand straight out and put the white slip of paper even with Stan's eyes.

"In your face," I said, my annoyance evident in my voice.

Stan took the slip calmly from my hand and studied it closer then looked up at all in attendance and stated, "Yep, he got it."

Matt took the white slip and looked back at Stan.

"We know! That's what he said." Matt stopped just short of saying what everyone else was thinking: *You idiot!*

At least that's what I was thinking. Stan wasn't anything more than a warehouse man like me and the other thirty men in attendance. He was not a supervisor. My license status and the utilization of it had nothing to do with him. Stan just needed to know I had, in fact, achieved my objective—or needed to bring into light that I might have been lying.

I had asked around the warehouse the past month if any of my coworkers who were trying for the Class A license wanted to study. No one did.

After my truthful declaration of success, I realized I was the only one who attempted to reach for it. I was the only one to receive it. And the lead man, Stan from the grip department, was nowhere to be seen before the week was out, maybe due to his lack of diplomacy that brought down the team's morale.

Three days later a voice over the intercom called out, "Knight! Come to the supervisor's desk."

As I approached the desk, I saw that it was the warehouse supervisor, Rusty, a good guy, jovial, with bushy red hair.

"How would you like to do a beer commercial?" he asked.

"Yes!" I replied.

I was instructed to pick up a five-ton grip truck already loaded with huge lights and colored diffusion. I picked up the truck at four in the morning and drove it forty miles to Long Beach, California. I pulled into a commercial bar, but through city permits, it was the crew's for the day. I asked at one time if I could help with the lighting, or grip part of the commercial production, as standing around was never my forte, and was told no, as it was a union gig.

So I did nothing but stand around for the day, and then I helped shelve lights and cable. After I hooked up the generator, I drove the forty miles back, all for what ended up being $735 take-home for one day. I remember thinking, *Not bad for breathing in and out—that, and driving.*

Movies, videos, and more commercials, and soon enough I, too, could receive my union card. Don't get me wrong; it was a hard-ass job at times, and my longest day was twenty-one hours. I owned a new car, a street motorcycle, and a dirt motorcycle.

I had an apartment and a bank account that did nothing but grow. I worked almost every day, my pager never silent. After the word got out to other movie-production-rental houses, I was getting calls two and three times a day for production driver. This was well received by me, and it was all due to my effort and achievement of obtaining my commercial driver's license.

2

Driving under the Influence

One February night in 1992, I was invited to a friend's bachelor party. I did have one drink, refused the second because I was going out with another friend for dinner, and said I'd be back to finish out the night with them. I pulled out of the club in my fire-engine-red Camaro and hit the freeway. Aware of my surroundings, I saw there was a highway-patrol car left and to my rear. He was in the fast lane; I was in the slow lane, and everyone else drove between and past us in the middle lane. I signaled to exit, and the cop hit all his lights, crossed over three lanes, and pulled me over. After all the questions and Texas two-step moves, which I passed, the officer asked me to ride back to the sheriff's station with him. I thought this was strange, as was his benign, monotone wording, but also he was young and inexperienced. No cuffs were placed on me. I wasn't put in the backseat; I rode up front in the passenger's seat. He even left me alone when he went into the minimart, at least a hundred feet away, to tell the guy behind the counter that I would be right back for my car. All very peculiar. We got to the station and walked in casually, almost like when I drove an ambulance. We were like partners. I was a test subject for him to practice on. He led me to a room, more like a good-sized broom closet, of brick. The officer nicely asked me to have a seat. He briefly explained about a machine, a breathalyzer. It was a beige-colored box with a clear tube at one end and a small window illuminated green with a digital counter that read 0.00. I was instructed to hold the mouthpiece, and I blew into the breathalyzer and received a reading of 0.09.

A 0.08 or less and he'd have taken me right back to my car. As this wasn't the case, I received a DUI. I recall the officer slumping in his chair with more of a surprise on his face than on mine. This meant no more driver's license of any kind for an entire year, as well as the job that went with it. In short, I lost everything. That is to say, all things material as my ambition was fully intact.

Still legally able to drive for another forty-five days, it was my hope that I could work every one of those days, but within a day my "good friends" made it a point to tell others about my misfortune. One friend even drove to another of the equipment-rental houses just to relay the message, knowing full well what would happen. For the first time, my pager fell silent, as did my friendships.

3

Question of Ethics

had my day in court. Now, if I screw up, I'm the first one to say I did it! With this being the case for the DUI, I pled guilty. You're pregnant or you're not, you did or you did not; there's no gray area. I had a female attorney, Debra Blair, appointed to me. She was in her mid-thirties, approximately six years my senior. She was plain, but I attributed that to her lack of attention to her appearance. Had we been going out on a date, I would have said she'd clean up nicely. But the day-to-day routine of courtroom protocol caused some complacency on her part. Her charcoal-colored, white-trimmed blouse was not pressed. I'm sure it was nicer and more complementing a year prior. The blouse was buttoned to her neck with only the top button undone.

She wore a black knee-length skirt. Except for a pleat on one side, it was unremarkable. Her skin was pale, and I don't believe she got out much during the day to allow any time for the necessary exposure to the sun.

I pictured a drab office in her home, lots of papers and law books. At least one coffee cup with its accompanied spilt-coffee ring sat on papers of pending cases or the unfiled past cases of redundancy. Like the coffee cup, she just shelved both till another day.

Her legs were firm, and her skin in general was fair and clear. Her shoes were open-toe white pumps. A scuff here or there, but clean enough, and the most complementary items she had donned that day. It was as if she spent her entire morning on her choice of shoes. We were sitting in a small gray-carpeted cubicle between many others that lined the walls of a large room in the courthouse. Her chair was rigid, no swivel, no recline.

She crossed her legs elegantly, one knee over the other. She was poised, back straight and head up.

I thought for a moment, *Maybe she served time in the military.* Perhaps the phrase, "Stick out that chest, soldier!" had been shouted in her face a few dozen times. Whatever the cause for this posturing, she had it down pat.

In the actual courtroom, after a couple of legal mumbo jumbos, a caveat, and an addendum, all was done in court. Ms. Blair asked me to follow her, and she would direct me to where I could pay the fines for my misdemeanor indiscretion.

"It's on the second floor," she commented.

Through a courthouse foyer, she walked two or so feet in front of me, fumbling with some paper work. We approached an elevator with a small gathering of others waiting.

She sighed. "We'll take the stairs."

She spoke coyly and led the way. Halfway up the stairs of oak and cold, poorly decorated concrete covered in brownish carpet, she stopped. She turned her upper body left while holding the oak banister with her right hand, which brought her right knee in and her heel off the floor. Her eyes gazed downward over the rail, and she nibbled on the far-right edge of her lower lip as she collected her thoughts. Then she looked unwaveringly in my eyes.

She said, "I don't know how ethical this is, but I find you very attractive and would like to see you in another arena."

She handed me her attorney's card upside down; it had a penned-in telephone number in black ink. The numbers were pressed with disciplined attention, like the legal documents, as if this, too, was an area where it was, or was not, going to happen, and she was far too busy for gray areas. I knew now that what she fumbled with writing while walking to the elevator had nothing to do with work; this was premeditated pretension. She had moxie.

I stood with my right foot up on the next stair, my left hand on the same oak banister. I held my right hand up, and she handed me the card—a Shakespearean scene. She smiled a pleased smile, more an exaggerated smirk. She turned her head and threw her wavy blond hair over her right shoulder and proceeded up the remaining stairs.

A couple thousand dollars and a handshake later, I walked out of the courthouse more confused than when I went in.

I thought, *Life is whimsical.*

As I walked into my uncle's house, I saw my aunt sitting in the living room watching some banal television talk show.

She asked, "Did you get a DUI?"

I replied, "Yes, and I got a date!" I never did call the lawyer lady.

4

EMT—1A

explained to my uncle, "I won't fare very well sitting on my ass for a year." With a quick thought, I opted for something in the medical field.

Now, some years before the movie industry, I did receive my emergency medical technician (EMT) certification. I was in charge and drove a critical care team (CCT) ambulance for two years on the streets of Los Angeles, Hollywood, and the San Fernando Valley. But the sad truth is that saving lives doesn't pay very well at this end. I knew even then I'd have to increase my medical training if I were to equally increase my earning power.

It was very educational though. Injuries of every type, in abundance.

I remember driving south on the 405 freeway. It was about nine in the morning. I saw a light from one of the interior lights in the back of the unit. I asked my partner to go back and shut it off. He went back and shortly returned, but looking in the rearview mirror, I saw that the light beam was still streaming through.

"The light's still on, James," I said.

"It's not a light in the ambulance, Will. It's a bullet hole two feet behind your head. The light is from the sun on your left, rising from the east," James explained.

Well, that and a few other reasons were enough for me to execute a permanent leave of absence.

5

Nursing Endeavor

My uncle did the normal thing he usually did and gave a nod of approval with my medical-endeavor request.

"A nurse! Not an assistant. A nurse!" I said.

I went down to the career institute in my hometown of Simi Valley, California. I was raised there, and for the first six years of my life, I had ambulances in the driveway of my home. My father managed and ran the first ambulance service in our small, scarcely populated valley. So I guess it was in my blood by association. The Ronald Reagan Presidential Library would one day be built atop Mount McCoy, which was just outside our front door, west of our house, and behind a white Christian cross that rose above our valley floor.

I applied for the nursing program and found out shortly after that two hundred others did as well, resulting in a class of thirty. I asked the assistant director of the program, Mrs. White, what the length of the program was, and she replied eighteen months.

I thought to myself, *Two years!* "Is there any other way to complete the program sooner?" I asked.

Mrs. White replied, "Yes. There is a full-time course that will take nine months."

So I chose the latter of the two options. Then I was told I first had to complete a prerequisite, their Anatomy and Physiology class.

This would be my second time taking this class. I knew this would be a testing ground for all aspiring nurses, respiratory therapists, and x-ray techs. The powers that be wanted to see how well we did with attendance, attitude, and grades.

6

Anatomy and Physiology

The Anatomy and Physiology class started, and the instructor, Sandra, was a very nice woman in her late thirties. She had dark-brown hair and was fairly attractive. She spoke of this class's expectations of us, her academic crew.

In a louder voice, to establish a no-nonsense approach, she stated, "This is an eight-week course. You, however, have only six weeks to complete it!"

This only justified what I had already been thinking: *Who was up to the mark, and how bad do we want this?*

Most of my classmates gasped and looked around, but I just looked straight ahead and thought to myself, *I've done it before. I'll do it again, faster.*

We didn't know, yet, if we would make it into our respective classes of choice, and I knew this was where they'd weed us out.

The books were passed out and looked familiar. I'd seen them before. I also used much of the anatomy part to assess and explain many injuries involving bones; blood; and gray matter, or brain, as well as the symptoms of heart attacks, strokes, and diabetes, to name a few. I learned the workings of these organs or, in some cases, the lack of workings. Physiology played its part, and well. There were many days of study ahead nonetheless. Lots in fact. We arrived to class at eight in the morning. Class lasted till noon. After class my friend Richard, who was going for respiratory therapist, and I got something to eat and went directly to his house to study. We didn't finish till midnight. I didn't mind the hours of study. Richard was attempting anatomy and physiology for the first time, and teaching him helped me stay razor sharp. I recall Richard was having trouble remembering the lower-leg bones, the two below the knee (the patella). I've often come up with analogies to help myself recall things in the past. He had trouble with the tibia and fibula.

He said, "I get confused about what bone comes first."

I told Richard, "I will kick you in the tibia for telling me a fibula."

It was late, and we were tired and laughed generously at the educational humor. A good ending to a long day. The next day it was a final on the skeletal system, the naming of all the human bones.

I heard Richard laugh under his breath. He sat just in front of me. I knew he was naming the lower-leg bones just below the patella. Almost every day, the class had a final on one body system or something relative. The class was a blur. The last day quickly approached. Grade day. If not for missing one day because of the flu, I would have passed with an A.

"You deserve it," were Sandra's words.

She explained to everyone in the class that it would be at least two weeks after the class ended before anyone would actually know if he or she had gotten into his or her primary course of choice.

The last day was a hot one in midsummer in Southern California, where the air was almost too hot to inhale. We were sitting in the classroom, which was dark because the overhead lights were turned off. The sun was almost at high noon and streamed some light through the classroom door, which was open for air movement. We were watching a film on isotopes. The classroom phone rang, and the instructor, Sandra, spoke quietly and briefly from the far-left side of the room. Hanging up, Sandra tracked back across the room to my right. Ducking down slightly in the glare of the TV screen, she turned right.

As I sat at my desk, Sandra walked down the aisle—down *my* aisle.

I sat in the very back of the class; I didn't care to have anyone sitting behind me.

She walked past and behind me and then leaned in to whisper in my left ear. She said, "Congratulations, you just made the nursing program."

Her right hand was on my right shoulder. Not a pat on the back; this was softer. And as she moved away, her hand moved intimately from my right shoulder to my left shoulder. Unexpectedly, it raised the hair a bit on my neck, almost like some tango dance move, something I didn't put a lot of thought into at the time.

I was still thinking, *Watch what you ask for—you might get it.*

It would be a couple of months before the nursing program started, and some apprehension crept into my stomach. I sat staring straight ahead, but I could feel the eyes of inquisitiveness from my classmates moving over me like the reminiscent hand only moments before. I was quite inert.

At the end of the class, the instructor revealed she was having a traditional party at her home in Thousand Oaks, California, for all of us who survived with a passing grade. Now, I wasn't the oldest or the youngest. At twenty-nine I was somewhere in the middle. Some were housewives who desired to do something personal with their lives now that their kids were grown up enough. I applauded them for this undertaking—real enthusiastic go-getters.

From nineteen to forty-five and in between, there were equal numbers of male and female prospects for the medical field.

Ambition, anxiety, and confidence were a few of the ingredients for success in any endeavor. We all shared these mixtures.

Many of us accepted the party invitation as it would be good to cut loose a little after much studying and testing.

A couple of the guys from the class rode with me to Sandra's house. It was a large, sprawling one-story home, which looked to have about five bedrooms. There were no pictures of family to speak of. No kids. Mostly friends, with Sandra smiling for the camera in another part of the world—one shot showed the Eiffel Tower lit up in the background. No men's shoes or jackets. The house was tidy, and there was no dust where one might notice a picture, or pictures, had been recently removed in haste. The house smelled of chicken, recently cooked. Walking through the glass slider into the backyard, I saw no tools or large, heavy gloves laid over the edge of a wooden workbench. Instead, I saw a nicely laid out buffet of pasta, chips, and the aforementioned chicken. Off to the far right of the house were some small gardening supplies, potting soil, and empty plastic pots of different sizes. Sandra's backyard was large with a nicely manicured green lawn. Sparse, uniform rows of colored flowers accented the edges meticulously. Cypress trees lined up along the backyard perimeter, giving absolute privacy. A clean, clear-blue pool of more than adequate size dominated most of the yard.

Along the right side of the pool was a nice-sized Jacuzzi with a redwood lath gazebo that gave more privacy.

Three large, healthy, green ferns hung down from the gazebo, spaced in equal increments.

Candles of red and amber yellows, set in candle holders of different heights, dimly lit the interior of the gazebo; with the sun setting in the west, their brightness increased.

They must be new, I thought, since there was no long, hanging, melted stalactite-looking wax, which there would be had they been lit any nights prior. The Jacuzzi could accommodate about eight adults and enthusiastically bubbled in anticipation.

I thought for a moment, *Where's the guy now? He must have really fucked up 'cause it looks like she got everything in the divorce.*

Maybe I was being cynical; maybe she won the lottery or inherited the property from her Westlake, California, lawyer father.

But then I thought, *No! I'm a realist. It is what it is; he lost big time.*

I sat two bottles of wine on the bar, red and white.

Wine glasses were set on the bar as well as cocktail glasses and bottles of popular hard liquors and beer in ice.

Maybe the man of the house was just a tidy guy himself. I kept my apartment immaculate, too. He'll probably walk in any moment, I thought to myself.

Just then a row of yellow amber electric lights lit up around the pool area. I flinched a little, shocked out of thought and back into reality.

"Did I surprise you?" A playful voice said behind me.

I turned and looked.

Sandra had just shut an outside lighting panel after turning the lights on. Here, her hair was dark and hanging loose as opposed to in the classroom, where she wore it up.

Well, it was always damn hot in the classroom, I thought.

Smiling, I said, "Maybe a little. The place looks great."

Sandra replied, "Thank you. I try." Emphasis on "I."

She had on a lightweight white dress shirt worn open with a bathing suit top of ocean blue with yellow-flowered print lined in black, which reflected the yellow mood lights. It looked Hawaiian, and from the pictures in her house, it probably was.

"Drink?" she asked.

"Excuse me?" I replied before thinking, *Damn! Flower prints.*

She picked up one cocktail glass. I saw another glass to the left of an ice bucket. The glass had pieces of melting ice in it with a diluted clear fluid.

She's started drinking already, I thought.

Her back to me, the shirt she wore ended, and her tan thighs began.

"What's your pleasure?" she asked.

Smiling with closed lips, like I was holding back a laugh, I wanted to say, "What's your game here?" Like maybe she lured unsuspecting students to her lair, got them drunk, and seduced them. *I'll play*, I thought.

I replied, "I like potato juice."

"Vodka it is," she shot back.

I thought, *Oh, she's good, quick, downright pithy.*

Sandra had informed us that swimwear would come in handy, and for the most part, all complied and either brought or wore their swimsuits under clothing of light summer dresses or shorts, myself included. It was a beautiful, warm Southern California summer night. Splashes of tonic in drinks went with splashes in the pool.

It was quite apparent that I wasn't the only one who had the view of an anatomy and physiology book for the past one and a half months as my only company. It was like being a kid again, and the parents were out for the evening.

Let's see what kind of trouble we could get into, I thought, and I felt myself smirk.

The night went on with an all-around feeling of a theme-parks excitement. The temperature of the Jacuzzi was, of course, that of a hot bath.

I sank in slowly to allow an acclimation from cool pool water. The water flowed over my tan shoulders.

Ah, I can die now, I thought.

With no shortage of participants, the Jacuzzi was festive.

Sandra sat directly across from me in the circular Jacuzzi of undulating bubbles and hot opaque water. The steam rose and the sun had gone down a few hours earlier.

The candles were the only light. Silhouettes flickered about the gazebo in the red and yellow glow. A cozy, shadowy scene that was all too familiar, not being my first rodeo, metaphorically speaking. These nights and their recipe of water, heat, barely clothed anatomies, and shots of liquid courage on the inside would verbally manifest in the morning as excuses. The regular defenses of having had too much to drink, the favorite one of denial, and on occasion an accusation of one trying to blemish one's reputation. An accent of anger applied to the denial theatrics.

Immersing my entire body under the water, resurfacing with my head back to allow the water to slick back my dark-brown hair, bringing my hands over to strain the excess water, I sat back and rested my head on the concrete curve of the Jacuzzi, which could have been a feather pillow, it was that comfortable. I felt great. Warm water leaping about my neck and around all my companions.

Just then, the unmistakable feel of a deliberate foot on the inner-upper side of my left thigh. I opened my eyes without lifting my head. I knew who it was. Sandra and I exchanged a glance that confirmed what I had already known was the objective of "the game." Yes, this was far from my first rodeo.

In these arenas I can feel at ease. It's appropriate to play when both are consenting.

Not one time during the class was there any unwanted or suggestive misbehavior. I could deal with this. It's the lack of professionalism in settings requiring one to focus on why one is there that I have difficulties with. Especially if it's at the expense of another person, when that person is relying on one's training and sincere concern for his or her well-being.

My traveling companions to the party had left some time earlier, as did other former anatomy and physiology classmates.

Flirtations between Sandra and me gave way to body brushes and hand-to-hand nonverbal agreements.

"Spend the night?" she whispered close to my ear. Like she was reliving two days earlier in the classroom.

"Will I wake up to a less-than-enthusiastic man standing over me?" I jokingly replied.

"No, there will be no man, enthusiastic or otherwise," Sandra said, smiling a bit and in that confident tone she used the first day of class.

So the teacher kept me after the party for in-depth tutoring of anatomy and physiology, twice.

7

Entrance Interview

At my nursing entrance interview, for part of the evaluation process, I sat in a school chair. In front of me were two previous "star" students of the nursing program and Mrs. White, the assistant director of the nursing program.

Mrs. White was a fairly nice-looking Filipino woman between forty-five years of age and menopause. She was about five feet five with olive skin and straight black hair that came around her round-featured face and ended sharp at her shoulders.

She attempted to appear confident, but her occasional shy demeanor stood out long enough to shadow her futile attempts. She began the interview with the first question.

"What do I mean by being the patient's advocate?"

"The middle man, a voice for those who may quite literally have none," I answered.

She smiled and scribbled on her notepad as the other two interviewers asked me questions, too. All the following questions fell into the category of common sense, and I answered accordingly. How strange and ironic that the first question, which I answered short and sweet and perhaps most honestly to my character, would be my undoing.

8

The Nursing Program

I received my book list, which resembled the inventory of the Library of Congress. It wasn't that intense, but long enough—a list of reading material that made me wonder if I should have opted for the two-year nursing program. That thought came and went just as quickly, giving way to encapsulating confidence.

I'm in, bring it on! I thought.

The first day of the program came quickly. The instructor passed out a collection of handouts and folders of materials that included some strange lettering, lines over single letters, three and four letters in a row of no discernible meaning (e.g., "gtts (drops)," "prn (as needed)," and "npo (nothing by mouth)").

Must be a typo, I thought.

Then looking at the top of the page, I read the words, "Medical Terminology."

I thought, *Chinese or maybe one of the Philippines' languages would be easier to learn.* It's best to take one day at a time—little bites of knowledge as opposed to trying to digest everything in a day.

Live tomorrow when it gets here, I reminded myself.

So day faded into day, and the program had the momentum of a steady-moving freight train with no ability to slow down. Each week we turned in papers on whatever body system or disease was required. We received, or rather bought, uniforms that were white and pressed and resembled military uniforms. They had blue-lettered patches on the right shoulder, which creased with the sleeve, and name tags on the right-upper chest with our names engraved against a white backing. The letters were the same color as the blue patch with SVN at the end of our names (for student vocational nurse). The last two days of the week were clinical. We worked the floors of the hospitals, starting IVs, giving shots, and sticking catheters into every orifice of the body and some man-made stomas (orifices).

I had absolutely no personal life as I took this endeavor quite seriously. I broke up with a nice hometown girl whom I dated for close to two years, and I gave up Wednesday-night poker with the boys. In my mind I had shit to do—got to do it 100 percent, get it done, know all that was set down, ask in detail any question that applied, answer any question of me equally, be the best or get the fuck out and make room for one more worthy of this endeavor. Don't be a loser was my short and quick of it!

These references were paraphrased ways of how my father, an ex-military cop who served in Okinawa, Japan, would direct me most of my life. A strict man—patience was, as I recall, never on the top of his list.

I recall walking in from school one day at the age of fifteen. I remember the age because I walked; on my sixteenth birthday, I received my driver's license and bought my first car for a whopping $189.

As I entered our two-story dwelling, commonly referred to as a home, my father sat at the formal dining-room table studying real estate or astronomy, which he received his associate's degree in. At this time he was already a paramedic with the Los Angeles City Fire Department. I don't know if it was a reverse-psychology tactic or vindictiveness, but I was greeted as I entered the house with, "Loser's home!" It was a comment I brought up years later as I read many books on psychology and had excelled in the subject since high school. I wasn't looking to blame or play the poor-poor-pitiful-me card. He emphatically denied ever remembering saying it, and he said if he had, he apologized for it. A sincere remark, he meant.

Back in Anatomy and Physiology, I met a girl who would later bear me a son—more on that later. She, too, made it into the nursing program. As I like the back of the room, the first three days were like musical chairs, a pairing up, everyone breaking off into his or her own tribes of two or more.

On the third day, it was Alexis and me in the very back left-hand corner of the room. Alexis was nineteen years old but intelligent, mature, and independent. I might be ten years older, but she seemed a little more grounded than I was. An anchor I could moor myself to.

She was very quiet in speech and manner, petite with a well-balanced figure. She had brown straight hair past her shoulders with bangs that fell just above her brown eyes. When she'd smile, it was grand and drew me in closer. Her full lips glistened with gloss that contrasted with her straight bright-white enamel finale. Our peers guessed quickly that we were involved. I didn't even think about age, and she never said anything.

Since there were two clinical hospitals, fifteen nursing students would go to one and the other fifteen students to another. Alexis and I went to the head director, Mrs. Harris, and asked that we be split up. Alexis could go to Ventura Community Memorial Hospital in Ventura, and I could go to Los Robles Hospital in Thousand Oaks. This was received by Mrs. Harris very well, and she said it was a very mature decision on our part.

Mrs. Harris was an African American woman of maybe fifty-eight. She frequently stated she was approaching "the age of purple." I didn't have a clue what that meant. Her hair was black and kept neatly styled, resembling a military beret. She held a demeanor of self-importance about her, and I still don't know if it was her personality or an aura that went with her educational background. I believe maybe a little of both. With Mrs. Harris's permission, Alexis and I were to go to different clinical hospitals. The fact was Alexis lived in Ventura, and I lived in Simi Valley. This allowed us more time for activities of daily living and to study, and it was less distance to travel as well.

Both in the clinical hospital setting and with ourselves, we honestly wanted nothing to distract us from becoming competent nurses.

Time was slipping by, and we all seemed to be evolving into nurses and regressing from ourselves, like a military platoon acting as one. Patient care is something I've always done and will continue to do with utmost respect. It's something I pride myself on. We were still technically student nurses, but the people we cared for were the real deal with normal apprehensions and fears of the unknown, asking me on occasion what I knew about their prognoses. The law is, though, that we nurses, or students, couldn't give answers that were above our scope of practice, our level of training (LOT). These pieces of information, good and bad, were left to their doctors.

With each accomplished task, treatment, procedure, or paper came a sigh of relief. The next hurdle of medical academia lay in wait and made me hold my breath.

The first day we were to administer medications arrived. Here, the human body can receive medications via many routes, determined by the medication, its intended use, and the patient's ability to swallow, and all avenues would apply. With medications come risk; that's a given. To decrease the risk of medication error, one should know as much about the medication as possible. I'm sure I'm not wrong in this principle. Pharmacology is an ever-augmenting creature that demands one's respect.

I had been working with about five patients on the med-surg floor for approximately three days. I knew medication administration was eminent. I had written down all of their medication regimes with a pen that holds four colored inks. I studied what the med was, what it did, where it did it, side effects, contraindications, all of it!

With my head looking down at my medication sheet of rainbow colors of red, black, green, and blue ink, I stood alone by one of two medication carts. They rested at the wall inside the nurses' station that divided the two hallways. The nurses' station was quiet, except for the occasional patient bell that would buzz till a nurse or certified nursing assistant (CNA) answered it at the patient's bedside and silenced the alarm with the push of a button. In the nurses' station were books; procedure manuals; a *Physicians' Desk Reference* (a drug book the size of *Webster's Dictionary*); and nursing drug handbooks, which are smaller, personal nurses' drug books that could be, and should be, carried with nurses to any floor, like their stethoscopes.

In the station was also a sink of white porcelain and a stainless-steel paper-towel dispenser that sat above the sink, waiting for the fiftieth time you would need to wash your hands. To the right of the sink sat a red "crash cart," hardly a term of endearment. The crash cart was used when a patient was found to be in full arrest, or in serious respiratory or cardiac distress leading up to death.

That's when you would hear "code blue" and the room number three times in a methodically calm, drawn-out voice.

"Code blue room one twenty-three, code blue room one twenty-three, code blue room one twenty-three."

Without changing tone, it could easily sound like an announcement over the hospital intercom speakers, as if someone left his or her car's lights on in the parking lot.

On the crash cart's side was a red sharps container of used needles, bearing a hazardous-materials logo on the front. It was accompanied by another equally ominous-looking one that hung from the wall.

Nurses who worked in the hospital came and went, as did attending doctors, showing up like uninvited guests to write an order, check a lab, or just sit and stare in thought, like they had just returned from the front lines of battle. That "thousand-yard stare." They all had it occasionally— Doctors, nurses, and now me, I realized.

I stared down hard and studied my medication sheet. I looked at the medication I was to give first.

Mrs. Harris walked in to the nurses' station where another student and I waited, my classmate at one medication cart and me at the other. She walked around the station with no apparent destination or task, just filling space with her presence. She paused and then approached the other student to my left. I heard Mrs. Harris speak to the female student giving her first medications.

"What's the name of your first medication?"

The student nurse answered and gave the name. With all medications come two names; these are called the generic and trade name. Mrs. Harris didn't ask for the trade name of the drug.

"What is it?" Mrs. Harris asked.

The student replied, "I have no idea."

Mrs. Harris and the student nurse began to laugh to the point where they both had tears in their eyes. Recomposing themselves, they talked about it briefly, and Mrs. Harris told the student, "Give your med."

Now it was my turn. As Mrs. Harris approached me, the director's smile faded, and her demeanor changed to one of no-nonsense.

"Mr. Knight," she said as she stood next to me.

All four of the male students in the program were addressed formally with "Mr."

I acknowledged her. "Yes, Mrs. Harris."

"Are you prepared to administer your first medication?"

"Yes, Mrs. Harris."

"What is your medication to be given?" she continued.

"Lasix."

"What is its generic name, Mr. Knight?"

"Furosemide."

The questions conveyed faster.

"What is it?"

"A diuretic."

"What kind of diuretic?"

"A loop diuretic."

It was becoming more like a game show than a hospital, and the clock was ticking.

"What does that mean, Mr. Knight?"

"That this medication's action is realized within the loop of Henle."

"And that can be found where?"

"Located within the kidneys."

"What is the medication's purpose?"

"To reduce the volume of body fluid, any excess of water."

"What electrolyte does it deplete?"

"K—potassium, the intracellular dominant ion."

"What's the extracellular dominant ion?"

"NA—sodium, and Lasix inhibits its absorption."

"If there should be an imbalance of either of these electrolytes, what could be expected if not corrected?"

"Arrhythmias, an irregular heartbeat, which could be fatal if not corrected or supplemented with one or the other electrolyte. Deficiency of either electrolyte will show on the individual patient's blood lab work."

Just short of asking me the inventor's hair color and his or her mother's maiden name, she responded.

"Mr. Knight, what are the five nursing steps?"

I went blank. A mental fog had abruptly rolled in. I recalled a decade ago I forgot how to spell the word "is." It happens, I guess.

When I focus as hard as I was and am thrown a question out of the blue, I need to reboot, if you will, for the category and application.

"I am unable to recall this at the moment, Mrs. Harris." I surrendered.

"That's a red flag, Mr. Knight!" Mrs. Harris replied.

Red flags were bad. I heard them in circles around me but never had one red flag addressed to me. Till now.

This question and the answer was something the class went over months prior at the beginning of the semester. I couldn't recall the answer. My mind was 100 percent focused on not killing someone, this being the first day of medication administration. As she continued with the seriousness of the question, I found her walking slowly into my personal space, and I backed up accordingly. I then realized I was no longer in the nurses' station and was at the fire-escape exit on the third floor of Los Robles Hospital. I stopped and put my hand up with a straight arm.

"Hey! I don't have an answer for you at this time. You want a paper written on it? A short novel?" I exclaimed.

I knew she could see by the look on my face that this conversation had reached its end.

"OK, Mr. Knight, return to the nurses' station and give your med," Mrs. Harris said.

I brought this question up to another student mere moments later, and she replied, "ADPIE!"

I remembered the acronym instantly: assess, diagnose, plan, implement, and evaluate. I recall thinking, *We use this every day as a nurse. It's our blueprint.* It may have been either in the way she asked or my intense desire to memorize all the medications, but the fact was, the director was going to continue asking me questions till she found one I failed to have an answer for. I felt like I just underwent a cerebral enema.

The following Monday I was called into the director's office. I walked out of the class and along the concrete corridor, dodging other students from other medical classes. It was a sunny, warm, breezy fall day with strokes of white clouds surrounded by blue skies.

Simi is a Chumash Indian word meaning "wispy white clouds." My hometown's namesake was in full dress. Daydreaming, I found myself walking up a concrete, handicapped-accessible ramp to Mrs. Harris's office, a brown building of dread. Mrs. Harris's green door was open. I stepped in. Mrs. Harris rounded her desk and began to tell me her reasoning for her persistence.

"I like to push my students, Mr. Knight," she said.

Something I was acutely aware of. At this point I wanted to say, "Can we quit this shit with the Mr.?" My female classmates were addressed by their first names.

"It's just I'm finding it very difficult to find anything to push you on," she continued.

"Then stop pushing me," I retorted.

"You tend to get animated," she said, standing close and eye to eye with me.

"No, I tend to get pissed off," I retorted again.

I calmed myself with her equally calming retreat.

Push didn't come to shove.

"OK, Mr. Knight, you may return to the classroom," she said.

I think being in a warehouse full of men sweating, cussing, and throwing things in anger and watching minor fights fueled by a couple after-work beers had left my edges in need of some smoothing.

It was and still is my opinion that Mrs. Harris got off on making the female students cry in hallways by bullying them. Listening to her condescension, I coined the phrase, "Education by intimidation and humiliation."

The days and nights of homework, lectures, clinical settings, papers on diseases, care plans, and case studies continued. Procedure day, we were taught about the nasogastric-tube (NGT) insertion. We used a mannequin of sorts that gave a transparent view of the inner workings of the human throat, including the esophagus, stomach, bronchioles, and lungs. The tube is inserted through the nose (naris) down the throat (esophagus), and into the stomach. One of the reasons for this was to empty the contents of the stomach so a doctor could perform an endoscope, the insertion of a small camera that can help uncover the cause of a gastric bleed or can provide a general inspection of the esophagus and the walls of the stomach.

9

NGT Stat

The assistant director, Mrs. White, who took over my clinical rotation, approached me on a medical-surgical floor in a somewhat urgent nature.

She said, "Mr. Knight, we have an NGT insertion in the ER, stat!"

For anyone not in the know, "stat" means right now!

The normal approach was to allow the student, me in this case, to overview the procedure first and then proceed. But this wasn't the case for me, confirmed by Mrs. White's statement: "And you don't have time to look over the procedure." This further justified my belief that this was a witch-hunt, that they were looking for me to screw up. Looking for my Achilles' heel.

I pulled my stethoscope from the side of a medication cart and proceeded to follow Mrs. White.

We went down three flights to the ER. I asked for the patient's chart. It was here I'd find the doctor's order in detail. I approached this elderly woman of approximately eighty-five years of age. She was frail and thin, normal for the most part. Her pallor allowed her veins of blue easily visible just beneath the paper-thin skin that covered her forearms. She was alert and calm, and she seemed to appreciate the attention. Again, a normal aspect of a geriatric setting. I knew she arrived from a nearby convalescent hospital, as stated in her patient history in the same chart, of course. I find it interesting how the human species would be happier that something bad or ugly was happening to them as opposed to nothing day after day, or months if not years, long periods of time alone with nothing more than memories of a life lived as company. I saw this in my first clinical setting of geriatrics. I witnessed it enough to know I was making an educated observation here.

"Hello, Mrs. O'Donnell," I said with a slow and calm approach.

"Hello," she replied with a soft smile. She seemed to trust me and feel safe. I smiled back and leaned on the rails of the bed, a more personal feel than just moving about the area like she was a third person in a two-person play. To put her more at ease, I used some small talk and stated how cold the ER rooms were kept. This would allow me to know how cognizant the patient was to her surroundings (person, place, and time).

I then introduced two of my fellow female students to the patient. Mrs. White stood silent and observant about five feet from the foot of the bed. I advised the patient that the other students were here to assist me in the doctor-ordered procedure. Both students stood by quietly, maybe even a little hesitantly. I then asked one of my student-nurse counterparts to take a bath blanket and put it into the microwave for twenty seconds, turn it over and run it another twenty seconds. I had the other student nurse get a cup of water and a straw. The blanket that was warmed in the microwave was returned, and I pulled the drape that hung around the individual ER beds; its metal glides swooshed in a circle, closing off the rest of the ER and world beyond to provide the patient with privacy. I explained to the patient that I was going to remove her blanket and sheet. Then I would place the warmed bath blanket over her and then replace her original covers. This would alleviate the coolness I'm sure she felt as it was somewhat cool for me as well. The lady smiled when the warm blanket was unfolded and laid over her, followed by her original blankets.

Mrs. O'Donnell commented, "That's much better." A clear verbalization and proper response.

I do things like this out of common sense. To gauge patient awareness. To encourage the patient to verbalize his or her needs. And I do for them as I'd want done for me. I change places with the patient and think about how

I would like to be treated—respectfully. This is a lesson that most medical professionals would do well in remembering.

Having gone over this procedure in class, I began.

I explained to the patient that I needed to place her in an upright sitting position called a full Fowler's position. After the patient smiled and nodded in understanding, I proceeded. I explained in full detail what I was going to do and for what reason I was doing it. As I placed the tube up the nose, some pressure was to be expected when it reached the back of the throat (nasopharynx). Turning the tube, which was lubricated, clockwise just a little, the tube slid down. One student assisting me held the water with the straw in it up to the patient. Taking small sips of water through a straw helps facilitate the tube to be directed into the stomach. The tube was measured from the ear to the nose and just below the xiphoid process (sternum), which gives a good measurement of "placement," as the tube could deviate from the esophagus and go down the trachea into the lungs via the bronchioles, causing respiratory complications. After placement was checked by taking a sterile 60 cc syringe of air and depressing the plunger of the syringe and osculating, or listening to the patient's abdomen with my stethoscope, I could hear the bubbling sounds of the stomach's contents. Then, per the doctor's order, the tube was hooked up to a longer clear tube to a vacuum at intermittent suction. I turned on the machine and received an instant return of 500 cc of frank—or visible—red blood.

I remember thinking it looked like a kid's crazy straw with cherry Kool-Aid swirling up and around like a roller coaster.

The vacuum receptacle hung on the wall just behind the patient's bed. I was glad about this, as it may have caused her undue stress. The sight of that much blood at once could unnerve anyone, especially if it was your own.

The procedure was done per the doctor's order, and the area was cleaned, and the patient was made comfortable. I then told her what was going to happen next with the endoscope, and that unlike the past when surgery was needed to fix an ulcer, it was now cauterized with a laser.

"Then you can be made well faster and get us out of your hair and return back home." I spoke in a joking manner.

The elderly lady smiled and placed her left hand on mine, which rested on the chrome steel rail of her bed, and said, "Thank you."

I put my other hand on top hers and replied, "You're very welcome."

I recall thinking, *I'm happy I was the one to do this for this lady. Where she was afraid, I was able to comfort. Where she was cold, I was able to warm. Where she was sick, I was able to help in facilitating her well-being.*

This feeling of contributing to another—*maybe being a nurse wasn't going to be a substitute. I may have found my calling,* I thought.

After charting in the nurses' notes, the other two students and I were instructed to return to our respective floors by the assistant director, Mrs. White.

"Mr. Knight," Mrs. White called to me as we walked toward the exit of the ER. The two other students continued on.

I turned toward Mrs. White.

"Yes," I replied, and stopped.

"Mr. Knight, I must say in all my years as a nurse, I have never witnessed a more complete execution of any procedure. You had the patient's trust, and you explained very well what you were going to do. You saw to the patient's needs that go with observation, and you didn't look up to me at any time for assurance."

I knew the reason for this part of her statement. Other students when administering a shot or catheterization looked up at Mrs. White, or another instructor, for assurance, nodding their heads up and down as if to say, "Is this the right way?" This lack of faith in one's abilities causes an equal lack of trust from a patient, and some embarrassment for the instructor.

Mrs. White continued. "I have never seen a more professionally complete procedure from a doctor, nurse, or student. I'm truly impressed." Her enthusiasm covered her normally shy manner.

"Thank you very much, Mrs. White, but I can't take all the credit. If you recall, it was you who taught us this very procedure in class. I paid attention." I smiled.

With her coyness returned via a smile, Mrs. White looked down and then back up. "You may return to med-surg." She excused me.

10

Halfway There, the Blue Stripe

The months passed and graduation was approaching. At the sixth month, the halfway mark, we had an assembly at the Simi Valley Library.

We were to receive our "Blue Stripe," something like a military rank for those who made it thus far. Some recognition awards were handed out to a few, including myself. I don't recall the others, but my award was for "Most Congenial." Other words for this are friendly, good natured, hospitable.

Pictures were taken afterward, and some refreshments were served as families met and talked with each other. An all-around good day.

As my uncle drove me home, he said, "Halfway there!"

I was glad to see the smile on his face. It wasn't there because he was the one who paid for me to undertake this endeavor. It was a proud smile. He knew what I was going through. He'd awakened me on more than one occasion at three in the morning, asleep at the computer. My efforts did not go unnoticed.

Things between my classmates went very well, as did things with my girlfriend, save a bump here and there as in all relationships.

I recall one day, Maryanne, one of my fellow nursing students, was standing in the hall just outside of pediatrics, and she was crying. I knew that Mrs. Harris had made her rounds and bullied Maryanne into tears. I walked over and gave her a hug, and she rested her head on my chest and wrapped her arms around me. In other settings of this kind, it would have meant a mandatory meeting in the parking lot or hallway with the "bully." I was still working on smoothing my edges. We were to be professionals here.

That kind of mentality was inappropriate. It's just too bad Mrs. Harris, our head director, wasn't aware of this. Maryanne was a Filipino girl of about twenty-three years old, maybe five feet three, black hair, and very friendly. Maryanne had a sense of mischief about her. She had explained that she didn't know some of the inoculations that were the norm in pediatrics.

"Didn't Mrs. Harris go over them with you?" I asked.

"No," Maryanne replied. I went over the medications and years of age each med was spaced, as well as boosters and the like. I left her smiling with her head up as she reentered the pediatric unit.

Mrs. Harris, zero—me, one. But the day wasn't over yet.

Coming in the mornings to clinical, we met in an office where we'd get our assigned floors. I was assigned to "post-op" this particular day, a station where people (our fathers, mothers, sisters, brothers, and us, God forbid) go for observation, where people go after having just been cut open to save their lives from one cause or another.

Again, we medical professionals would do well in remembering this fact—that we, too, are on the menu of life.

One nurse, who worked for the hospital, and I were the only two manning the post-op station. I went around and got familiar with the area and picked up Band-Aid wrappers and other pieces of trash. I unwrapped the EKG wires that were tangled, made up a bed or two, and went and sat next to the charge nurse.

"What do you do when there are no patients to attend to?" I questioned. Her reply came by handing me a book. She smiled. "They come in and go out, and in between we amuse ourselves."

Holding the book, I saw that it was titled *The Firm*. I did not open the book. At that moment Mrs. White leaned in the station's door, almost bent over. It looked like she might have been in a hurry, and she almost passed the door but remembered just in time to grab the handle. With just her left shoulder and head in the door, she looked around the room and at us, smiled, and just as quickly left for other floors requiring her attention.

Three more months and we who remained would graduate. A few of the students were dropped, or dropped, from the class. Being that it was none of my business, the reasons are theirs.

11

Baby News

A normal day around the homestead. The phone rang. I picked it up. "Hello! You Stab 'Um, We Slab 'Um Mortuary. We have our own rent-a-hearse, you haul. This is William," I joked.

"Not funny," Alexis commented. Her voice calm and steady as usual.

"Hi, honey. What's up?"

Alexis replied, in a matter-of-fact tone, "I'm pregnant."

"How'd that happen? We only did it once!" I said jokingly. I continued. "You need some pickles and peanut butter?...Hello?"

Alexis replied only with the sound of her breathing.

"I'm sorry. You just caught me off guard is all. Pregnant, really?" I asked.

Alexis's mother, listening in on another line, said, "You bet your ass!"

"My ass is fine. It's my ovaries that are killing me," I laughed.

Alexis just said, "We'll talk tomorrow morning, OK?" And she hung up.

Now, ladies, please take into consideration the fact that you are usually the first ones to know this, and we men are busy in our heads with school, jobs, mortgages, and remembering your date of birth.

So if we hesitate a moment or three, it's just that we need to catch up with this significant life-altering fact, so be gentle, please.

Being a nurse and exposed to all the floors of a hospital, I know it is very important that pregnant women should avoid some of these floors as they might be detrimental to the pregnancy.

At the beginning of this course, all the students were made aware of this fact, and if any women become pregnant during the course of the program, this needed to be communicated to the directors and instructors for safety reasons. In this arena keeping such a secret was not possible. If I was to become a father, then so be it.

The last three months passed pretty much uneventfully. That is to say, no outstanding moments of drama, and I am not complaining. The day of graduation grew very near. Our confidence in ourselves had grown; we were sharp and we knew it. My girlfriend, sharp and pregnant, took on a very angelic glow. She was beautiful.

12

Final Grade

I t was about four days before we walked the stage to receive our diplomas, get pinned, and say our oaths. Each clinical rotation was instructed to meet at five o'clock in the morning at a prearranged place. My clinical group of fifteen was to meet at Coco's Restaurant in Thousand Oaks. This is where we would find out if we passed the nursing program. An amalgam of the full year's grades would decide the final grade. We all knew we had passed as something would have been said already in words or in grades we already received after the many tests. A student or two had dropped the program, or the program dropped them. We were just going through the formalities. Today we would find out our ultimate grade and exchange mementos of pen sets and things like that to our clinical instructor, Mrs. White. We all had been through much in the past year. Literally, blood from the patients, sweat, and tears from the instructors as well as us students. There were still fifteen students in our clinical rotation; we didn't lose one.

We sat at tables that had been pushed together and aligned the entire west wall of Coco's Restaurant. Menus with colored mosaic-looking pictures reflected the gold of the early morning sun. Smiling and excited in our achievements, we reflected back in kind. We said good morning to one another sincerely, no forced pleasantries, no patronizing tones. We meant it today, and it was. We ate breakfast, laughed, and spoke about the upcoming state nursing boards we had to pass. We spoke of study groups, and most volunteered their homes. Others pointed out that the motels we were to stay in would serve as a good place as well to refresh our knowledge before the test. Our class would be the last class to take the written test for the state nursing boards.

The written test gave way to computer tests that maybe after seventy questions answered, the computer would shut off, leaving the results of how well they answered to the test taker while waiting absolution. Our written examination was held at the Pomona Fairgrounds. *There must be a thousand people in here*, I remembered thinking. There were to be five hundred questions to answer. *Or five hundred questions I could miss*, I thought. It's normal to be anxious, I supposed. Everyone else was. Still, as new nursing graduates, we had been tested and baptized under the florescent lights of every hospital floor and scrutinized by our nursing-program drill instructors. We would be fine.

It was ladies first to receive their grades; only three of the males in the class including myself were here.

One at a time, they walked through the restaurant. A sea of smiling, amiable faces of onlookers, themselves having breakfast. Happy rhetoric from other classmates filled the restaurant. Through the large, clean windows, I saw the traffic, heavy with Friday morning commuters on the 101 freeway heading into Westlake then on to Los Angeles to the east and Camarillo, Oxnard, and Ventura to the west. Classmate after classmate came back in the restaurant with euphoric smiles. Some with tears of accomplishment in their eyes. I was very happy for them. It was coming down to the last of my classmates, two males and a few females.

"William, you go!" my classmates strongly encouraged me. I walked the gauntlet of smiling patrons through the restaurant and came to the front doors of glass and pushed them open. Cool morning air flowed around me like cold water splashed in my face that opened my eyes wide from early morning squints.

I saw the desk that sat in the green grass left of the walkway. The assistant director, Mrs. White, sat on a formal chair behind it. Something about her manner didn't feel right with the overall cheerful atmosphere of the day. I pulled out the chair on the other side of the desk and sat down.

"Good morning, Mrs. White," I said affably.

"Good morning," she replied.

I thought, *There it is! That patronizing tone.*

She straightened the white sheets of paper in front of her in an uneasy, awkward way. She looked up and we made eye contact, and then Mrs. White looked back down in avoidance at the papers.

She said, "Mr. Knight, I'm unable to give you a final grade at this time as Mrs. Harris needs to speak with you."

It was like it was all the air she had left in her lungs, and it all came out in one full breath. She glanced to her left and never did look back up at me.

Coward, I thought.

I stood and pulled the chair back. Now I was unhappy, to say the least. Maintaining my professionalism, I apologized to her for any inconvenience I may have cost her this morning. I reentered the restaurant and walked back to the tables. I didn't want to take away from the exuberant mood of my classmates. I didn't know what to say.

The proverbial rain on their parade, I thought to myself.

I smiled a little, but I was sure I didn't do a very good job of it. That old high-then-low mental crash. "I just have to speak with Mrs. Harris next week," I said.

I attempted to convince my classmates all was right with the world, and by their faces I knew for the first time in at least a full year, I failed miserably.

In support, I remained till the others received their grades. Looks of curiosity and confusion from classmates fell upon me like a cheap suit that made me uncomfortable.

I left alone, drove my car east a mile, and glided around the interchange from the 101 to the 23 freeway north. I went back to Simi Valley with a void feeling and little reality to grasp except a tangible steering wheel. The traffic had lightened up. I left the radio off.

I went over scenarios in my head of possible shortcomings on my part. Reasons why the program's hierarchy denied me this day of all days escaped me in total. I thought of what I'd tell family and friends who waited in Simi Valley as well as other parts of the world. Everyone knew about this day, even a couple who hoped I'd fail the program, their effort to maintain their illusion of master.

As I drove I drifted in thoughts that took me some years back, just before going to Pierce College for my emergency medical technician certificate (EMT-1A). I had briefly worked for Ford Automotive. My friend Ron, who worked there for a few years already, had brought me in. I knew it wasn't what I desired to do for any length of time; I required a bit more *ad* in my *ventures*. I recalled sitting in my bedroom at the foot of my bed. I was wearing a white dress-uniform shirt with Ford insignias. I was almost twenty years old. My father walked down the hall toward the garage door and noticed me sitting there.

"Aren't you supposed to be at work?" he asked.

"Yes," I replied. "I guess."

I sat physically indolent, but mentally I was in full vigor. I was looking down at the brown shag carpet.

"I need to do something else." I spoke this thought out loud.

"What do you have in mind?" my father asked.

Standing up, I grabbed my keys. "I don't know," I said as I walked past him. "I'll see you later." I walked out the front door.

I drove over the hill east on the 118 freeway (the Ronald Reagan Freeway) to the San Fernando Valley. I exited De Soto and headed south to Roscoe Boulevard, where I worked. I didn't stop. I ended up in Woodland Hills. I turned left. A marquee stood out high in the air on the south side of Victory Boulevard just east of De Soto. Behind it spread out Pierce College, a large campus. I pulled in and parked. I changed into a shirt I had in my car and walked in, still having no academic direction. I walked into the office where pamphlets were stacked. Above them a sign read Class Courses. I picked up a pamphlet and flipped through it. *I'll know it when I see it*, I thought. And then the words "EMT-1A" hit me like a slap in the face. An almost embarrassingly obvious choice. Between two and nine years old, I grew up with ambulances in our driveway—late-night emergencies with red and blue lights racing across my bedroom ceiling in circular motions. My father was a Los Angeles Fire Department paramedic himself.

I'm so mentally myopic was my self-chastising thought.

I obtained the necessary papers and found the class.

This class was full; at least twenty people stood around the back wall of the class. One of the two instructors spoke at length.

"Most of you will not be here after today, so I'll allow everyone to remain at this time."

Odd, I thought.

Books were passed out and opened. Pictures of dismembered bodies, blood, brains, bone marrow, and cerebrospinal fluid, to name a few, immediately started to thin the academic herd. One person, and then three people, walked out; some appeared to have an appointment to revisit their previous lunch. I remained in my seat and looked down at the book. *Interesting*, was all I thought.

I guess the engrossing, in-depth stories my father relayed during spaghetti dinners, detailing eviscerations with intestines strewn out, desensitized me a bit. Everyone had a seat before the end of the first class, with at least three more to spare.

I drove back down De Soto north toward the 118 freeway after the class ended. I turned left on Roscoe and right on Owensmouth. I parked and went into Ford to tell my manager about my set intentions. I walked through the showroom, down a hall, and into Mr. Brown's office. I apologized for my absence and explained myself. He intently listened, a nice break from the norm for him.

"That's great!" he replied sincerely, and shook my hand. I recalled feeling hope from his sincerity that there was still hope for the human race, in that rarely you came across one who genuinely wished you success in your endeavors. I thanked him and walked back into the parts department where my friend Ron worked.

Radiator hoses and fan belts hung about the place, smelling of rubber.

Large books of part numbers littered the room. Ron, overhearing my conversation with the manager, walked around the long parts counter, dark with years of grease stains. He was straight faced with a hint of concern. He placed both hands on my upper arms and looked me in the eye.

"Don't do it! You'll be back in two weeks begging for your job," he said.

There was an urgency one might hear when being told not to jump off a forty-story building. I looked down at his hands, left then right.

"I don't share your doubts, Ron. This is just the start," I replied.

The master syndrome again. Was he really concerned about me losing my pedestrian job? Or was the thought of me achieving higher prestige one that apparently scared the hell out of him?

Six months later I graduated. After passing the EMT course, I moved out of my father's house and into Wood Ranch at the far southwest corner of Simi Valley.

I drove the critical care team (CCT) unit five days a week, twelve hours a day. I lived with my girlfriend of three years at the time. She was a former Miss Simi Valley. She was beautiful, intelligent, and funny—still with a trace of vulnerability, I recalled.

After almost a year of driving the ambulance, Ron and I were speaking over margaritas, like nights before. He admitted that my success in getting my EMT had left him envious. He was renting a friend's childhood bedroom, from the friend's parents, still pulling auto parts, which was fine, I guessed. But the justification of my thoughts of his fear of my success were realized.

About eight years later, it was just before the start of the nursing program. It was Wednesday-night poker. A friend, Carl, held these games at his house. Carl was about ten years older than everyone else, a nice guy and fair host. Among the regulars were Ron (from my brief Ford job and also a friend I'd known since kindergarten) and his two younger brothers: Richard, who took the Anatomy class with me and failed to get into respiratory therapy, and their youngest brother, Jerry. With two other male friends of ours we sat at a formal dining-room table, playing any game of cards that had "poker" in the name.

The conversation fell on Dan, a fifty-something former poker player who lost his house when he was laid off from his job and had to head up

North for work. Carl, Ron, and Ron's brothers passed a white sheet of paper around that resembled a football betting pool with dates like a calendar and initials in boxes. Ron asked me if I'd like in.

"What's the game?" I replied.

"It's not a game. It's where you try and pick the day when Dan fails and comes back," Richard said in an obtuse tone.

"You're betting that another person will fail?" I asked.

"Yes. It's two dollars a box, and if he doesn't come back in a month, we're going to use the money for a barbecue," Richard explained.

"No, betting on someone failing is not my thing," I stated with an overtone of repulsion. It's the first time Richard was absolutely right: it wasn't a game.

"Then do you want in on the one we have when you fail out of the nursing program?" Richard asked, smiling.

Every head at the table turned and looked at him with strong stares of "Shut up!"

Richard broke the silence. "I'm just kidding," he said, and shrugged. But the damage was done, and everyone knew it.

This was the last Wednesday-night poker game for me.

My thoughts returned to the present, and I found myself driving east on Tierra Rajada. Caught up in thought, I didn't remember exiting the 23 freeway just south of Moorpark.

Entering Simi Valley, I drove down Los Angeles Avenue, turned right on Fifth Street, and then left on my uncle's street and into his driveway. He and my aunt sat in lawn chairs drinking coffee, both smiling. A beautiful Southern California day. The dark-green leaves from fruitless mulberry trees shaded the driveway. A feeling of dread filled me. If not for a degree of indignation to balance me off, I could go as far as saying I bordered panic. I parked, got out, and walked up the drive.

"Well?" my uncle asked.

I replied, "Oh! I have to wait till Monday. Mrs. Harris needs to speak to me first."

My futile attempt again to persuade a status quo. The smiles faded.

"Why?" he asked. We all knew my grades. I never missed one class. I could only say I knew as much as they did. So I was to wait the weekend before I was told my academic efforts might have been in vain.

Monday arrived, an overcast day, the dreary morning gray.

Perfect! I thought.

Few classmates sat in their seats. Everyone was smiling and looking forward to graduation. I held little part in what should have been a happy day for all. I looked around the classroom at full-body mannequins and transparent half-torso replicas of the human anatomy. A five-inch blue string hung down from one of the chalkboards that used to have nine white nursing caps with the names of the past nine months on them. They were cut off one by one by a different student each month, signifying progress. I saw it as a countdown. Stethoscopes and blood-pressure cuffs were neatly placed on tables along the back wall of the room for the upcoming class of students.

I don't envy them, I thought to myself.

Classmates sat atop desks and talked. This was the day we were informed about the upcoming graduation. One of the five lecturers and procedure instructors, Mrs. Smith, walked in the classroom door. She was maybe sixty years old and the most pleasant, down-to-earth lady I had ever met. There were no airs about her; in a word, she was compassionate. This softened me a bit. I was anticipating Mrs. Harris. My patience exhausted, I wanted the wait to be over.

The classroom phone rang and answered my prayer.

"Mr. Knight, Mrs. Harris would like to see you in her office," Mrs. Smith said, her voice so kind. I softened even more. With a nod I stood and, collecting my book bag, felt all eyes on me. My girlfriend, Alexis, placed her left hand on my right hand as I stood, looking up at me with a small, white smile of encouragement. I smiled back and leaned down enough to place my left hand on her stomach. She put her right hand on top of mine, and we paused for the cause. Moments earlier I was reassured by many of my classmates that all would be fine as well.

John, one of my classmates, said, "You helped half of us pass this class." Other classmates in his company nodded and smiled in agreement. I did help many of my classmates, but they helped me equally.

I walked out of the classroom and down the hall of concrete that lined the outside of the buildings of red brick. The walk was covered by a tin overhang and held up by green poles in increments of about twenty-five feet apart. I was used to walking in clusters with my classmates, but now it was deserted and quiet and had aged, a long-ago feeling. I passed through a patio of tables with steel, connected benches, where we all used to eat many lunches over the past year. This, too, had turned into a ghost town. I could almost hear echoes of past conversations, laughter, and tears. A chain that locked the school's perimeter gates clanged in the distance on a steel pole with the occasional breeze and broke the silence. Looking ahead, I saw the familiar brown bungalow. I walked up the concrete ramp, cold steel handrails on either side. I stood at Mrs. Harris's green door. On both sides of the door were tinted windows. I took a breath. I knocked. One moment, two, and then Mrs. Harris opened the door. She smiled enough to set herself at ease, but it did nothing for me.

"Come in, Mr. Knight," she said.

Her preamble, like many times all year, was to ostentatiously push her hair just above her left eye with two left fingers, slow and deliberate.

With a hand gesture to a chair opposite her desk, she said, "Have a seat."

I thought, *How quaint.*

I took the arm of the chair and turned it slightly to the right and slid in.

The chair had a black, five-inch padded vinyl cushion and back of equal size, with a chrome steel-structured frame.

Mrs. Harris's desk was oak laminated and neatly kept. Three pens were spaced an inch apart. Another black vinyl chair sat adjacent, with a high back on it, and it was swiveled out to the left. A few odds and ends were intentionally placed. There was a picture of no real purpose other than to show the color contrast of a brighter nature against the dark-brown walls. Mrs. Harris, in a self-aggrandizing way, sat in her chair and swiveled center with the desk. I put my book bag down on the light-brown, clean, indus-trial carpet. I sat straight, and our eyes met.

"Mr. Knight, I have some concerns that I wish to discuss with you," she stated.

Concerns are good. I can live with concerns, I thought.

"Your clinical instructor and assistant director, Mrs. White, has written me with a couple of things I feel we need to address," she continued.

For a moment I thought, *Is she going to reiterate everything? We'll be here another damn year. I know Mrs. White's title.* I grew irritated.

"Mrs. White says she had you perform a nasogastric-tube insertion in the emergency room at Los Robles Hospital," she stated, reading from a paper.

"Yes," I replied.

"Mrs. White states here, 'Mr. Knight is overconfident in his abilities.'"

I shifted a bit in my chair and clenched my teeth.

"She states here in her letter that she also witnessed you in post-op reading a book instead of attending to patients?"

I replied, "No, that is incorrect."

I put my hands together and leaned forward. If these were the reasons for not giving me my final grade, I was going to have my say, especially when I didn't get to exercise my right to face my accuser.

Mrs. Harris asked, "Would you care explain?"

"Yes, I would, thank you," I said with insistence.

Mrs. Harris looked up at me like she had forgotten six months earlier when I put my hand up in protest to her obsessive question about the five nursing steps, what she described as "animated." I, in turn, described it as "pissed off."

I then reiterated the story of the NGT insertion in Los Robles ER and the words Mrs. White said regarding the procedure of which she had spo-ken so positively. I do not know how she concluded I was overconfident.

I continued. "As for the book, I was not reading it or anything else when she looked into the post-op door. I do know that there were no pa-tients at all in post-op, and the book in question had just been handed to me by the attending charge nurse after a question I had asked. Mrs. White wasn't in the room long enough to draw two breaths let alone come to such a hasty conclusion."

Mrs. Harris sat quietly and alert.

"I also see these concerns are dated, so it would be no problem to find the name of the charge nurse through employee records, as well as the day's post-op patients, that Mrs. White states coincided with my presence."

Mrs. Harris looked down at the paper on her desk, regrouping her thoughts in response. "Well, Mr. Knight, I do have some concerns of my own. You did pass this program, and you will graduate," she said, as if to defuse the situation. It was at that moment I stood up. With a look of surprise, Mrs. Harris stood as well.

I began. "I know what I just did, Mrs. Harris. Standing up is viewed as an act of defiance." I was done with being her inferior. I heard all I needed to. I was going to pass. Her concerns were just that: her concerns. "Mrs. Harris, I read the book you wrote on professionalism. I do recall it coming up in class briefly. I spent personal time and read it completely. In my opinion to read your book was to read your mind and thought process," I vented. I might have pushed the envelope here. It was unclear now who was the authority figure and who was the subordinate.

Since the book was on the mandatory book list that each student, every class and every year, was required to purchase under the program curriculum, she sold many of her books.

I took a breath and collected myself.

I said, "Mrs. Harris, as nurses we may cross paths in a hospital sometime in the future, and I am very *confident* I will be able to alleviate any *concerns* you may have of me." I made sure I used the two words that defined my conviction. Picking up my book bag, I turned and walked out the door. Mrs. Harris said nothing in reply.

I walked a fast pace back through the patio area, down the concrete corridor, entered the classroom, and sat in my chair. Classmates now sitting in their chairs listening to Mrs. Smith looked at me with the obvious question: *Did you pass?* Mrs. Smith included, I assumed.

"It was all a misunderstanding," I said. "I passed."

The mood lightened. And I thought I felt the August temperature drop a few degrees.

"What did I miss?" I asked indirectly. I leaned down and pulled out a notebook from my book bag, angry to be used by Mrs. Harris for no valid reason, other than to play the "master syndrome" card on me one last time. It was a waste of my time as well as three days of undue stress for me. If I were to ultimately pass the nursing program, Mrs. Harris's and Mrs. White's invalid "concerns" were irrelevant, cruel, and unprofessional.

Mrs. Smith continued, and I quickly deduced the subject was the graduation rehearsal at the new Rocky Peak Church.

The next day the whole class met at the church, a most exquisite venue. There were oak walls all around and four full sections of seats divided by three large accommodating aisles. Recessed lighting in the ceiling illuminated a stage approximately five-feet high and took up the entire east end of the church. It reminded me of a smaller version of the Universal Amphitheater, in Universal City, California. We were choreographed from the beginning to the end of the graduation ceremony.

13

Graduation Day

The women dressed in their white pressed uniforms with new, bright-white traditional nursing caps. The men dressed in pressed white pants, white shirts, black ties, and white waist-length medical coats.

Each man wore a purple rose on his lapel. We appeared to have just finished a military-run nursing program. Except for mandatory push-ups, it wasn't far off.

Family and friends packed the church. Twenty-seven students. We sat in a row facing the stage as Mrs. Harris spoke about the past year, what we had endured. I was somewhat impressed by her detailed description; it humanized her. In five chairs on stage, set to the far left, were our lecture and clinical instructors. Prompted by Mrs. Harris, she asked us to stand. We all stood in concert. Mrs. Harris then introduced the vocational nursing graduation class of 1993, at which point we all turned in unison and faced our family and friends. It was a fine feeling to accomplish something of such a positive nature. It felt like everyone in attendance had their part in this aptly named *relative* moment. If it was to have only tolerated angry outbursts in frustration at home or rides to and from school or hospitals, this night was truly everyone's. The proud feeling overshadowed any animosities we, or I, felt over the past year.

Instructed to take our seats, Mrs. Harris and Mrs. White walked to the right of the podium centered onstage. On a white, covered table rested twenty-seven diplomas. In alphabetical order we sat, and in the same order, we were called one by one. The audience applauded each graduate. I could tell by a slightly more enthusiastic group per name that this must be the graduate's family of supporters. I sat third from the last, but not least. This chair was for my girlfriend, Alexis. She was radiant and three months pregnant, though physically it didn't show. After each took the stage, my name was called. The left half of the church lit up in cheers. So much so that every instructor sitting in the five chairs turned their heads with big smiles, some laughing. My parents, grandmother, uncle and aunt, brother, sisters, nieces, and nephew were sitting just behind me.

Also included were Carl from Wednesday-night poker, his wife, Ron, and both of Ron's brothers. Perhaps it was an attempt at apologizing, or a must-see that I succeeded. I walked to the left of the stage, climbed the eight or so stairs to the top, and walked back across to the middle. Heckling continued in short bursts from Ron and his brothers. Everyone quiet now, I turned toward the audience as instructed in rehearsal. Mrs. Harris presented me with my nursing pin, pushed it through my starched, white left collar. She then proceeded to give me a hug, one you'd expect worthy of a soldier returning from war. I reciprocated the hug in kind.

"We did it, Mr. Knight," she whispered in my ear.

Out of twenty-seven graduating students, I was the only one she hugged.

Mrs. White handed over my diploma with a disingenuous smile while again looking down and away. Two feet over, Mrs. Smith held out a scroll of white parchment, our nurses' oaths. She handed me a battery-operated white candle with a glass flame.

"Congratulations," she said, and smiled.

I put my arms around Mrs. Smith and hugged her, and she me.

"Thank you, Mrs. Smith," I quietly said.

My thanks to Mrs. Smith was for her humanity, her courage to be real, more than my admiration of her. I had never met an individual that held such a sincere and humble regard for one's neighbor. It was something of a comfort that told me there weren't only pretentious bitches and bastards strung out on power trips that went with wearing a name tag; there was also hope for mankind.

I walked to the right of the stage where the other twenty-four graduates stood. Rows of seven—it looked like the picture position in elementary school. I took my place. The last two grads were called. The lights dimmed. We turned on the switches on the bottoms of the candles, and their glass flames illuminated. A soft amber glow set a mood of seriousness. Mrs. Harris then led us in the reading of our oaths, our responsibilities as care providers, as medical professionals, and as human beings.

Finishing, we walked off the stage from the center. One after the other in reverse alphabetical order, in five-second increments. Down the middle aisle and out the church doors. It was done. My next thought: *now the California state nursing boards.*

With an overview of the nurse *National Council Licensure Examination* (*NCLEX*) book, an amalgam of everything we were taught in nursing school and should know, in questions with four possible answers, it was off to Pomona Fairgrounds for the written five-hundred-question test. It was like clockwork, literally, as we were timed. The test was taken and passed by all my classmates.

It's required of all nurses to complete thirty hours of continuing education units, (CEU) in California every two years. This amount of necessary CEUs depends on the state where you received your degree. Being an accredited nurse means you can practice in any state in the United States. Of course, after paying the necessary amount of money to the capital of the state you relocate to. California and New York nurses are required thirty units every two years. Other states require fewer CEUs, the lowest amount being six. If a nurse from any other state wants to practice in California or New York, he or she will be required to take the state's nursing boards first.

As new graduates we had four years before our renewal went into effect. So technically, we nurses weren't ever going to be done educating ourselves. This was to be expected. With the constant changes, new medications, and procedures, we had to stay sharp.

Weaned from the nest, only a few days after my boards, I applied and was quickly accepted for my first position as a nurse. All nurses who took the state nursing boards had to wait for their individual results. This wait could take up to a month, give or take. In Fillmore, California, I would make my nursing debut at a convalescent hospital, a geriatric hospital or skilled nursing facility. Obviously, there are different ways to address such hospitals, but unlike the names, the care was exact. It is a slower-paced hospital than the acute setting. Slower because of the longevity of stay for the patients, or, better phrased, residents. Residents of their last place—if coherent enough to know what their chronological, mental, and physical geography was, the realists knew this was the last place they'd call home. This statement is not one made from assumption but fact as I have had many residents confirm this verbally to me.

There are fewer admissions than an acute hospital. Still there were more falls, or acting out, to name a few, that would require incident reports detailing the situation. I aimed my sights for the acute setting, as did many others. I would have to wait for the opportunity. I settled into the routine of the hospital. I was a charge nurse for one of three floors. The hospital was shaped like a cross, with three patient floors and a floor for supplies, a day room, and a formal dining room. A foyer when you first entered the building held offices. One was for Mrs. Lambert, the director of nursing (DON), and the other for the administrator. The position I held as a charge nurse could be slow at times but could abruptly call upon one's total skills in an instant. Therefore, the unbroken routine did not go unappreciated. I recalled many nights to follow that the eleven-to-seven shifts were not the most coveted. I still don't know the cause of this. Maybe because I'm single, no wife and kids at home, nothing to answer to yet.

The norm for humans is to sleep during the night, which is a given. With patients, though, we nurses were 24-7. We knew this going in to this career, at least I did. On several occasions I was approached by my DON, Mrs. Lambert, a short, pear-shaped lady of fifty-five. She was a few pounds overweight and, for the most part, just going through the motions. Blond, yellowing hair hung about her shoulders. Due to a call-off, usually by the nurse scheduled for the eleven-to-seven shift, Mrs. Lambert would ask me to cover the shift after my own shift of three to eleven. This meant I would come in to work at two thirty in the afternoon and not leave till eight thirty the next morning—sixteen hours. Since I was already there, I don't recall ever turning my DON down. After the day's end, I would take reports from the other two floor nurses who were leaving. After the other nurses had left the building, it was only me for a one-hundred-bed facility, and the census, or number of residents, was close to capacity. I had four certified nursing assistants (CNAs) to work beside me. They were very professional in their duties, I remember. It was the CNAs' normal shift, and they had a routine set down that made for a smooth night. When I first started covering the eleven-to-seven shift, I asked all my certified nursing assistants to gather for a quick meeting. It was here I discussed my philosophy, my expectations, when it came to the residents.

I explained that I was not the boss. Yes, I was their supervisor but not who they worked for.

"We work for the residents," I said. "We're all licensed to a degree that makes us medical professionals, and our conduct should reflect this. I don't like someone looking over my shoulder, and I won't be standing over yours. We know our jobs, and now you know my expectations. Let's see to our duties and have a good night," I finished.

Yes, they were good, but I felt I needed to set the tone of who I was. I hadn't gotten to know them as yet. It served as a peace of mind for me. It felt like it did in elementary school when we took advantage of a substitute teacher.

We all did.

14

Anne's Alzheimer Dilemma

During a regular shift one evening, one of two other attending nurses, Anne, a young Filipino woman of maybe twenty-five, had a situation with a patient. Anne was tall and slim, pretty with pitch-black straight hair just past her shoulders. She was quiet, and I don't recall ever hearing her speak till this night. Anne had a patient in her charge with a diagnosis of Alzheimer's disease. This hospital was not a lockdown facility. At best the doors had alarms attached that would sound when the door was easily opened from the inside. Many of the residents could go in and out of the building at will, but through the front door only.

This patient of Anne's, Mr. Davis, was a white male of approximately seventy-five years of age. At about six feet four, he looked to be about 230 pounds. Not an ounce of fat on him. He appeared to have been in the navy at one time and was very self-disciplined. His arms didn't have the common atrophying appearance that comes with age. He had tattoos, one of an anchor with faded lettering, possibly the name of a ship he served on. He was strong physically, but his confused mental state, indicative of Alzheimer's disease, made him angry and hard to manage.

As he was Anne's patient, I took a second place to her and her responsibility for Mr. Davis, who demanded to leave the hospital.

Mr. Davis, adamant in his desire to leave, walked down the west-wing hallway toward the west exit. Anne walked behind him in what I perceived as a hope he'd forget what he was doing or where he was going. He didn't, and Anne attempted to take him by the arm and talk him out of his departure. Mr. Davis pulled his arm away in a manner that conveyed if Anne tried again, Mr. Davis might become physically confrontational—something Anne would be powerless to control, something I would have more than a moderate degree of controlling. I stood in the hall but kept my distance as not to exacerbate the situation.

At the halfway mark, I knew by Anne's body language she was out of options. Her shoulders dropped. She looked down and to the left, searching for a solution in her mind. I was a little disappointed at first that she had not asked for my help, but at the same time impressed that she hadn't. I walked to her right and passed her. I caught up to Mr. Davis trudging toward the exit. I decided I'd better try to supply a solution for Anne, who had all but given up.

I walked on the right side of Mr. Davis. I smiled.

"Good evening, sir," I said calmly.

"Evening," he replied.

"Are you going out here?" I asked.

"Yes, I am," he retorted. I felt the consternation in his voice.

"Great, I'm going this way, too. Do you mind if I walk with you then?"

"No, it'd be fine," he replied more softly this time but kept a hard eye on his objective.

I had about twenty feet to the exit door. I stepped a little faster.

"Let's go." I encouraged him.

Mr. Davis hesitated in his step.

I thought, *Pull, they push; encourage, they hold back*. A play on reverse psychology. I reached the door and disarmed the buzzer's combination. I opened the door wide and held it for Mr. Davis.

"Sir," I said, holding the door.

It was dark outside, real dark, especially just having walked out of the fluorescent-lit hallway. There were few lights at this time of night in Fillmore, a rural area really, with the location of the hospital set in avocado and orange groves.

It was a clear fall night, and the stars shone brightly because of the dark and lack of a moon. It was cold, and I used this fact to my advantage.

We both walked west down the sidewalk, away from the hospital, and I paused just enough to allow Mr. Davis the only choice of going right or left. He chose right, north to the main highway, 126, a major thoroughfare for eighteen-wheelers. I looked back a moment and saw Anne walking a small distance behind us. This was still her patient and her responsibility. I smiled, an attempt to reassure her. She didn't smile back. I kept a slightly faster pace than Mr. Davis, and it was obvious he was resistant in keeping up; he was doubting himself.

Conversationally I asked, "Where you headed this night?"

Mr. Davis replied, "I'm going down here to catch a bus, find a phone, and call my daughter to come pick me up."

I slipped my watch off my wrist covertly.

"A bus? What time is it?" I asked, holding my bare arms in what light there was from a lone streetlamp.

Mr. Davis was wearing his watch and looked down at it but was confused and said nothing.

"Is that eight o'clock?" I said, glancing over at his watch. "Oh, the last bus came by here at six. Won't be another till six tomorrow morning."

He looked toward the 126 highway in the dark and slowed his pace greatly. We were surrounded by avocado trees. The night was dark, cold, and damp. Mr. Davis had a cream-colored dress shirt on and no T-shirt.

"Well, sir, all I have on is this light shirt. I should've brought a jacket!" I commented. I didn't use the word scrub top or hospital attire. I didn't want him to remember where he just left and get his second wind. I rubbed my arms.

I stated, "It's cold out tonight. Winter's just around the corner. I'm going back. You have a good night, sir," I said as I turned away from him, giving him full autonomy of his decision.

Mr. Davis was standing inert, staring down the deserted street somberly. He took on a more subdued look; he was tired and it showed. I stepped back toward him slowly. I looked in the direction he stared. A dismal prospect ahead. Anne stood still and observant, ten feet away.

"You know, sir, I have a little pull over here," I said, looking around like I was doing something I shouldn't and gesturing toward the facility.

"I tell you what I can do. It's like a hotel here. I can get you a private room, you can get a good night sleep, and in the morning you can have breakfast and coffee. Forget the bus, I'll let you use our phone. Your daughter can pick you up right from here. Do you like milk shakes? Vanilla, chocolate, or strawberry? Hell, all three if you want. I'm the boss," I said, and smiled.

"Well, that doesn't sound at all bad," he said.

After a few more seconds of staring down the street, he turned slowly back in the direction of the facility. I didn't force the walk. I commented on being cold one more time just before the open door. The three of us walked back in. I showed Mr. Davis to his room, first one from the large nurses' station. I asked one of my CNAs to get me a shake, one carton of each flavor. I helped Mr. Davis with his night clothes from the personal items he was going to leave behind. I turned the TV on low with the news, just audible enough to make a distinct murmur. He dressed and lay down in bed with little effort. When I checked on Mr. Davis moments later, he had drunk two of the three shakes and was fast asleep. I turned out the light.

I returned to the nurses' station, a white-walled octagon. Close to one hundred patient charts filed via room number sat in racks against the back wall. Taking a chart of one of my patient's under my arm, I sat down and opened it and began to write my patient's weekly summary. I sat in one of three swivel chairs, and Anne sat in another.

Anne called Mr. Davis's daughter. She would be at the hospital first thing in the morning. The third nurse, a male about ten years older than both Anne and I, stood for a moment at the outer edge of the station, looking at each of us before he picked up some supplies and walked off. Anne looked over at me then away just as quick. She looked over a second time. I stopped writing, cupped my pen in my hand, and swiveled a bit to the right from my patient's chart and toward her.

I asked, "You OK, Anne?"

She put her pen down and swiveled a bit to her left. We faced each other.

"What are you doing here in this setting, William? I think you missed your calling. You should work in an Alzheimer's unit. I've never seen anything like that before. To influence with the elements. Knowing he was confused, you led him verbally, not physically. I'm glad I witnessed it," she said.

"Maybe, Anne, but do you know how mentally exhausting that would be after an eight-hour shift?" I replied.

She thought a moment and then looked out toward Mr. Davis's room. "I guess. You were so sure that he'd come back. How did you know?"

"I didn't. If Mr. Davis had continued to stay the course of leaving, we would have had to call the police and explained to them his diagnosis. He would have been taken to a lockdown facility," I explained.

"That would have been terrible," Anne said.

"I know. That's why I tried what I did."

"It worked!" she said, smiling.

"Yes, it did...tonight."

Anne and I spoke of many things this night. She was a very intelligent young lady. I thought back to many nights past, never hearing her speak. Now she spoke profusely, and I listened gladly.

15

Administrators' Deceit

Days and nights passed, and I worked five days a week, with almost three of those days double shifts. I worked Thanksgiving and Christmas, mostly because many, if not all, of the other nurses were married and had children. Family is important, and I found some reward in covering shifts that allowed them their holiday time with their families. As for my girlfriend, we had been enduring pre-baby turbulence off and on for months. I thought maybe it was hormones, but I didn't say anything. Some days were great, others, not so great. We didn't hold the monopoly on relationship unrest; it was just our turn, I guess.

Work was structured. I could count on the stability of it.

January was in the air and just a few days off the horizon. My director of nursing came to me at the nurses' station.

"Hello, William. I am in a spot. I have no one to cover the eleven-to-seven shift on the first of January," she said.

"You mean New Year's Day?" I asked.

"You'll receive double-time pay, like Thanksgiving and Christmas," she said.

"That's fine, Mrs. Lambert," I said.

I never put money as my priority. I thought of the night in question and the party my girlfriend and I were to attend, the pros and cons. The pros won. I agreed to cover the shift on the first of January. The choice didn't help me any in my relationship with my girlfriend. The night came, and in an hour it would be New Year's. The night was uneventful. I gave a report in the morning to three oncoming nurses and left. I drove the forty miles home over Grimes Canyon. It's actually a very scenic drive through avocado and orange groves. I applied at what would be my first acute hospital setting in Simi Valley. I liked the pace of an acute setting. A constant change of medications and diagnoses kept one learning many new things each night. Admissions, transfers, discharges, and the occasional code blue.

Doctors' orders seemed never ending. Observations and direct complaints of symptoms required skills on every level. I would wait for this opportunity a little longer. I continued working in Fillmore patiently.

Payday rolled around. Checks were passed out, and like always I just put it directly in my pocket and continued with the matters at hand. After my shift I opened my check and looked over my hours. A blank space in the holiday column caught my eye.

Where's my New Year's holiday pay? I thought.

I walked the rest of the way down the hall and into Mrs. Lambert's office.

"My holiday pay is absent from my check," I said, holding my check.

"About that, William. Mr. Gomez doesn't consider you full-time, so you don't qualify," Mrs. Lambert replied complacently.

I felt like I had in the movie-production warehouse seventeen months earlier.

Oh, those patronizing tones, I thought. "Well, Mrs. Lambert, you and I had an agreement. I don't care if I work one hour a week or ten thousand, till hell freezes over, you owe me a hundred bucks, give or take," I stated. "I work sixty to seventy hours a week here. I'm a full-benefited employee that only comes with full time."

I walked out of the DON's office and out the front door of the facility. Arriving home, I pulled out a folder and put the documents inside.

As nurses we document everything; we have to. I placed my pay stub in with the rest, taxes and such. Mr. Gomez was from Puerto Rico, about thirty-five years old. He was an obese man. He spoke very little English, and I'm being generous. He was the cousin of the woman who married the man who owned this facility and five others in the western hemisphere. It was Mr. Gomez's job to keep costs down, but now it was being done at my expense. I continued to work my schedule, and whenever Mrs. Lambert or Mr. Gomez came around the nurses' station, I'd innuendo around the hundred dollars in question. I had a lot of fun with this. It really pissed them both off. It wasn't so much the money as the disrespect, the lack of professionalism, that I found disappointing.

One day as I worked at my medication cart, Mr. Gomez walked into the nurses' station. He attempted to ask for something but made no sense as usual. One of the Spanish-speaking CNAs translated for him.

"He's looking for a four-by-four sterile gauze," she explained.

"Tell him it'll cost a hundred bucks" I said, and smiled. "Tell him that,"

She did, and Mr. Gomez looked up at me like always when I made these statements. Any time I could, I'd bring up the money, and I did it a lot. So much that my DON, Mrs. Lambert, and Mr. Gomez didn't frequent the nursing floors much anymore. It went on like this for a few months. I wasn't giving up. Meanwhile my application was accepted for the acute hospital in Simi Valley. I gave my two weeks' notice. Just like I thought, I received all eleven-to-seven shifts. I didn't care. I knew they wanted me as far away from them as possible. I granted their wish and counted down the nights till I went to my new position at the acute hospital in my hometown of Simi Valley.

Three days to go, and I drove the forty miles into work. I walked down the entrance hall into the nurses' station for patient report.

"What are you doing here?" asked Manjiet, a regular night-shift nurse. She was from India and was pleasant for the most part.

"I work tonight. It's here on the schedule," I said, picking it up.

Looking down at the shift in question, my initials had been crossed out and Manjiet's name was written above. She denied any knowledge of it.

"OK, then, good-night to you," I said.

The next morning I called into Fillmore and spoke with the DON, Mrs. Lambert.

"I came in last night and was told I wasn't scheduled. Since I was to work the eleven-to-seven shift and having driven to the facility, and the fact I was not to cover this shift was not communicated to me, law dictates you owe me for four hours," I stated.

"Please hold a moment," Mrs. Lambert said.

The phone clicked and then clicked back.

"Yes, William, you will be paid for the four hours, and we have the remaining nights covered, so you need not come in," she said.

"Oh, I'm coming in. Right now in fact. As soon as I hang up, I'm coming in. I want a check for my regular pay and a separate check stating holiday pay for the past New Year's Day," I retorted.

I heard Mrs. Lambert sigh heavily. I went upstairs in my apartment and retrieved a document. I drove to the facility in Fillmore directly. I walked into the hospital and into Mrs. Lambert's office. I was sure she was in no mood to talk as she handed me two white envelopes. I opened one. "Holiday pay" was written on the top of one of the enclosed checks.

"Well, it took seven months, but I got it," I said.

I thanked Mrs. Lambert and walked out the facility's front door. I opened the second envelope containing my regular pay. I looked at the document I brought from my apartment; this paper was a copy of the past two weeks' time card, electronically stamped. Looking at the card and at the check, I saw that they had taken eight hours off my regular time and used it on the holiday check. I drove down the street and made five copies of my time card and corresponding paychecks. Walking back into the facility, I first went to Mrs. Lambert's office.

"You will want to come with me to Mr. Gomez's office," I stated.

Mrs. Lambert labored around her desk and followed me accordingly. We both entered Mr. Gomez's office where he sat behind his desk.

"What?" he said.

I replied, "I won't waste my time here. You gave me my holiday check, but you took the eight hours to do it off my regular hours. Here's a copy for you." I slipped a copy across his desk. "Here's one for you," I said, handing it to Mrs. Lambert. "I'll give one to my lawyer, keep one for my records, and one for the California state labor board." The words had just left my mouth when an abrupt sound of a straining groan from Mr. Gomez's chair dominated the verbal silence as it rolled back, abruptly colliding with the office wall. Mr. Gomez stood up just as abruptly and leaned to the right where a wooded cabinet sat. He pulled out the facility's petty-cash checkbook, lifted it high, held it over his head, and with all his weight slammed it down on his desk. Yellow Post-its and pencils took flight in all directions, and most fell to the floor. Mrs. Lambert stood back a step and remained rigid in response and surprised at this angry, animated outburst.

"Pay attention, Mrs. Lambert, this is professionalism at its best," I declared with a smile.

Mr. Gomez then pulled out a calculator and punched away at it. He ripped the check from the book and thrust it toward me. I calmly accepted it.

After looking briefly at both of them, I just turned and walked out. I was disappointed that it had to end the way it did. I had good coworkers and good times. I learned much. With this day's unpleasantness behind me, I looked forward to my new start.

I thought to myself, *I'm off to bigger and better*; I was right about the first part.

16

Engaging

My girlfriend and I were set to continue our education and increase our level of training (LOT). And our baby was on the way. I thought, *This is it. I love her. She tells me she loves me. Now is the time.* We're both bringing half to the table of life. Both wanting to educate and provide a quality life for ourselves and our baby.

On a warm, sunny day in the San Bernardino Mountains, I walked casually into a jeweler's in Arrow Bear, California.

I explained what my intentions were to a gentleman behind the counter. "I'm putting the ring together," I said.

I looked through the different styles of wedding bands and picked a traditional-style solid one. I purchased the amount of gold. I watched as he poured the liquefied gold into the mold. The diamond I intended for the engagement ring I had picked out about a month earlier. The gold was polished to a fine shine. Then he set the half-carat diamond. It was a humble but excellent ring, appropriate for a beginning and a good foundation to add on to over time.

Things had been going well for us. I was looking forward to being a father. On a cool, sunny day we went to lunch at the restaurant El Patio. There was a winter-blue sky. Three evenly spaced evergreen ficus trees in one long, white planter that divided the patio. I suggested a seat at one of the tables under an umbrella. The restaurant wasn't crowded.

Holding Alexis's chair out, I asked "What do you feel like for lunch?"

"I think a chicken salad. It's healthy," she replied.

Always doing things right, Alexis was regimented. I stepped around the table and sat down. A waiter brought over two glasses of water and menus.

"A chicken salad. I believe that comes with a side order of willyoumar-ryme?" I said, like it was one word.

Alexis didn't get the meaning. "A side of what?" she asked, looking down at the menu as if to read what I said.

"A side of will you marry me?" I articulated.

She looked up instantly, taking it in to be sure. "Yes!" she replied.

Still nodding, Alexis began to cry. Her sincerity took up residence in my throat. I retrieved the blue-felt box from my coat and opened it. Inside was a brilliant-gold band supporting a diamond displaying a kaleidoscope of colors escaping their prism into the afternoon sun. Alexis was equally radiant. I placed the ring on her finger. We kissed.

We moved into a newer townhouse in Ventura. I had accumulated new furniture over the past year from moving in and out of apartments each time Alexis told me she didn't want me around. We made up the baby's room. I worked at two hospitals, and she worked at another. We bought new cars and one for her mother. One of the pantries was our own private baby Walmart. A few days later, I was asked by my fiancé if her mother could live with us. Her mother, a recent widow—Alexis's father had died months before—was a certified nursing assistant. I knew that Alexis would not have asked to have her mother live with us if it wasn't necessary.

Keep the peace, I thought.

"Yes," I said.

I knew her mother had reservations about me, having once called me a cradle robber in reference to Alexis's and my age difference. That, and she had said once I was egotistic. One day I was moving some boxes and wood planks that went with my king-sized bed for supports of the mattress. One plank had slipped from my grasp and fell flat on the hallway floor upstairs. *Slam!*

Both Alexis and her mother downstairs yelled up the staircase, "What was that?"

I replied, "My ego."

They both instantly laughed generously at my witty reply; it made me happy that I was able to bring laughter into our home even if it was humor directed at my personal character.

Time passed, and our baby was soon to be born. I recall being called at my uncle's house by Alexis's mother, Julie. I was told Alexis was in labor and to meet her and her mother at Ventura Community Hospital, the same hospital where Alexis had completed her clinical rotation for nursing. I started my nursing rotation there, but when permitted, I continued at Los Robles Hospital.

I stopped at a bakery and bought some fresh chocolate-chip cookies. I arrived at the hospital and went directly to obstetrics. I met with the OB nurses and donned some white scrubs. I was led into Alexis's room. Her mother and a close family friend, Maris, stood at the right side of the bed, farthest from the door.

"Good afternoon, everyone," I said with a smile.

Alexis's mother and friend half-heartedly greeted me back in kind.

"You're here?" Alexis questioned softly.

I was somewhat confused and surprised by her comment; there was distance in her voice. I got a feeling of imposing on them and the event as a whole. I quickly dismissed this feeling as it was my child being born; I was going to be a father today—any minute as a matter of fact.

The chocolate-chip cookies dominated the smells of the hospital room.

"Anyone for a hot chocolate-chip cookie?" I offered, glad I brought a peace offering as I felt the eyes of Alexis's mother and friend fall on me as if I'd done something wrong.

Holding open the box, I presented a dozen large, gooey cookies. Her mother and Maris both accepted. I pulled the cookie apart in halves, the melted chocolate chips strung across from side to side like a hammock. I brought one to Alexis.

"She can't have one of those. She's on Stadol! You two know this," the attending nurse said.

She knew Alexis and me from nursing school. Stadol was an analgesic used for pain.

"Of course, I'm sorry, baby" I said.

Alexis just complied in silence. I set the box of cookies on the counter across the room and refrained from partaking myself. I put a chair on the left side of the bed. I took a sterile white washcloth and wet it with a bottle of sterile saline. I patted Alexis's forehead and brushed her hair behind her left ear.

"Hi, baby, how we doing?" I asked.

"Can you not say baby, just for now?" she replied with some frustration.

"Of course, anything you want."

"I don't want to do this anymore," she said.

I felt very alone in my desire to protect her, and with nothing I could do, I endured my own helpless feeling that something was going to manifest here and that I was absolutely powerless to stop.

"Do you want to change places?" I quietly asked jokingly.

Alexis failed to find the humor in my attempt to lighten the mood. The door opened, and Dr. Martin entered the room, as did another nurse. A quick exam was performed.

"You're fully dilated, Alexis," the doctor said.

In Alexis's quiet mood, she just nodded. She remained quiet, and except for breathing, she never made a sound. I held her hand. She squeezed mine.

A few short efforts later, I said, "We have a son."

I leaned down and kissed Alexis on the forehead. "His name is Ryan William Knight!" I announced.

"Can I have one of those chocolate-chip cookies now?" is all Alexis said.

We went home. I would sleep with my head at the foot of the bed, where we set up our son's crib. I stayed awake and watched him breathe.

In my time off, I gladly spent every moment with my son. After two months Alexis started to avoid me in her quiet manner. I knew this from times before, and I knew the outcome. She was now sleeping in the baby's room. I opened the door as she was exiting.

"What's wrong?" I asked.

"We want you to leave," she replied with some resentment.

We wanted for nothing. We were set on a course to continue with school, to increase our degrees.

I asked, and knew it would be in vain, "Can I do anything?"

"No," she answered.

"Why?" I somberly asked.

"I wanted a baby, not a husband," she exclaimed.

"Why me?" I asked.

"I wanted to know what I was getting," she stated, and walked downstairs.

In one year's time, she would ask me back seven times. Each time, I'd move out of my apartment or house and try again, and the seventh time, she came back pregnant by another man.

"Well, the baby can call me Daddy, too," I said, without reservation.

Again she wanted me to leave. This time I had to tell myself, "This time for good."

17

Moving Acutely Forward

Another new apartment and my position secured in the acute hospital, it was time to move on.

Walking down the hospital hallway of pale-blue carpet and faded, institutionally green-painted walls, I approached the nurses' station of the medical-surgical (med-surg) overflow. Having worked clinical floors as a student and the long-term geriatrics facility, I felt little apprehension in my abilities. I walked up to the medication cart to hang my stethoscope.

"What about him?" a voice behind me said.

Looking around, I saw a mature woman of about sixty, Carol, with blond, yellowing hair in curls that sat idle on her shoulders. To Carol's left was a Filipino woman maybe thirty-five years old.

"What about me?" I replied.

Carol said "Oh! Tia's looking for a man."

Tia shifted with embarrassment in her seat.

She was an attractive Filipino woman, about five feet five with a slender build. Tia was the charge nurse, dressed in a set of ocean-blue scrubs. Carol, in civilian clothes, was the station's secretary. This was my first day.

"Looking for a man to give the patient report to?" I said, smiling and trying to keep things light.

The report was given to me professionally by Tia, and after, I'd describe the night as awkward. For the next few days, I would be on this floor with Tia as the charge nurse. Tia had flirted with me with eyes and smiles. She had done my patients' charting the last couple of nights, and this made me uncomfortable along with her occasional hand on my shoulder. I wanted to be nice, but I didn't want to feel obligated by her doing my job. Not even a week at my new position, and I was already contending with personal issues. This was not what I had imagined, or desired.

I thought back to the warehouse, trucks, and equipment—long days of cable dragging, checking lights, and ballasts, when all I had to deal with was my job, and not juggle the whims of a coworker. Tia spoke about this being her last night on the med-surg overflow. She had been covering for another nurse the past week. She talked about her home base of physical rehabilitation, just down the hall. I explained that I was hired as a "resource nurse" with my home base being the main med-surg floor. This meant I could be assigned to any floor in the hospital. The only floor I refused was OB. It didn't bother me so much, but I could tell while in nursing school, where I had been required to work every floor, that it made more than a few women uncomfortable. Even on the medical-surgical floor. I had walked into a patient's room and greeted a female patient approximately sixty years old.

I said "Hello, my name is William. I'm your nurse tonight."

"No, you're not!" the patient replied instantly.

I had no problem with this. My position was to care for people categorically. So, as in nursing school many times, my female classmates and I would switch patients to accommodate any and all of the patients' modest concerns.

I recall some of the female students in clinical would come to me and ask to change a male patient for a female one. One should not take the refusal of a patient personally, and I didn't.

As Tia and I sat in the nurses' station, I charted my nursing notes and made small talk. It was about fifteen minutes before end of shift, almost eleven o'clock. The halls were quiet, and the lights had been dimmed by turning out every other florescent. CNAs answered the occasional patient's bell. Tia finally got around to asking the inevitable question.

"Would you like to see me tomorrow? I'm off work and thought I'd go shopping and have lunch in Venice Beach," she stated.

"That sounds nice, and I'm off tomorrow, too," I said.

"I know. I checked," Tia replied.

This relationship started to feel a bit cloak and dagger. Tia checking my work schedule and planning around it felt a little presumptuous to me, even though I'd been excused by my son's mother and was now single.

"Yes, I would," I replied.

And I actually did have a level of enthusiasm. I had spent much time on the Venice Beach boardwalk. I liked the tourist crowds and their accompanying amalgam of different languages, arbitrarily walking in and out of the stores of sunglasses, T-shirts, jewelry, and fine bistros, enjoying wine and live entertainment in the form of soft rock or jazz bands. In Venice Beach after dark, especially during the summer nights of Southern California, there would be parties in some of the condos that directly faced the Pacific Ocean. All that divided the condos from the sand was a twenty-foot-wide walkway. There was music, drinking, and all sorts of recreational substances; pot smoke was thick in the air. There were some very interesting people, and I'm not referring to their intellect, although I'm not saying they were completely void of that. The eccentric nature of some just added to a free-spirit escape from the norm.

"Sounds fun. What time?" I asked

"Come by about ten and pick me up. We'll have breakfast there," Tia replied.

"It's a date then," I said.

Tia nodded her head and swung her stethoscope around her neck. She looked thoughtful and passed me, staring. "I know guys like you," she said, not looking directly at me as she meandered past.

"What does that mean?" I asked, a bit defensive.

"You'll need to take an HIV test," she boldly said.

Little gray area in the reason for that request, I thought.

A quick thought back to the movie warehouse, to sets and stages. No, never on a set, but maybe once or three times at a wrap party. This was surreal.

Inappropriate for this setting, I thought.

Then again, the Christmas party was months away, and she obviously didn't want to wait. I guess we were going to end up in bed, and soon.

"I'll pay for the HIV test," Tia said in a matter-of-fact tone.

"So I got that going for me," I said with disdain. "You've only known me a week. How can you be so judgmental of me? What should I think about you? It's starting to feel like maybe this is something you do a bit more than I do."

Tia's head just tipped to one side, like I said something that breeched dating etiquette. She remained quiet.

"Are you going to have an HIV test, too?" I asked.

"I already did," she replied.

I felt like I'd walked into a movie halfway through. I didn't know the beginning, but I sure the hell knew the plot: me!

"Fine, we're just going out for the day. We can get a blood draw later," I stated.

It sure left little room for romance. I drove over in the morning to the San Fernando Valley and picked up Tia at her house. I was relieved to see that Tia's mother wasn't accompanying us. The way it was going with Tia, I thought maybe I'd be married before sunset. The way she leapfrogged ahead of me at every turn, perhaps I already was. There were no surprises, and the day at the beach was just that. The next day, Tia and I walked into Dr. Carson's office just south of the hospital. I felt like I was going to a veterinarian to get my shots before my adopted master took me home. I spoke briefly with Dr. Carson, who appeared to know more about the situation than I did. Word gets around a hospital fast. We left the doctor's office with a script for a blood draw and subsequent HIV test.

We walked across the street and into the hospital, down the hall, and into the lab. If this was the norm for nurses' foreplay, it sure lacked romance. A needle stick with a return of blood that quickly filled the vial, and we're done on our end. We spent nights together, appropriately dressed, while waiting for the test results.

It was about eight o'clock in the evening, and I was working med-surg. It was a busy night with no distractions. Dr. Carson walked down the hall between patient rooms. He walked over to me.

"The test was negative. Congratulations," he said with a smile.

That night Tia and I had a late dinner of sushi. I didn't tell her the results of my test. If things were going to progress between us, I had to have some autonomy in the matter. A few weeks had passed, and I knew she knew about the test results. She said nothing, and that endeared her to me somewhat. I realized she just wanted peace of mind that should we be dating and should we become intimate, we would be safe in doing so. It was a true exercise in universal precautions. A few attempts by phone from Tia went unanswered by me, solely because I didn't own a cell phone yet. I was either at work or home, so I had no need of one. With hints of inconveniences from Tia, she handed me a cell phone—then a credit card.

"No, I pay cash. I only like to pay for things once," I said, handing it back.

"I may want something, and I'll pay for it," she replied, handing the card back. That feeling of being fattened up for the kill lay heavy in my stomach. I made little use of the phone, mostly speaking with her. As for the credit card, it went in my wallet and grew moss. Tia had asked me for items mostly when she was working and I was not. I picked things up for her but always paid cash. I didn't tell her.

On a rainy morning, we were sitting at Tia's kitchen table drinking coffee.

"Would you like to go back East with me?" Tia asked.

"Back East for what?" I replied.

"To see one of my friends in Virginia. I have the tickets," she said.

This relationship felt more like surfing. The wave picks you up, and you have no choice but to go with the flow.

"All right, back East to see your friend why?"

"She's getting married."

Tia already had the tickets. Again, she made plans, and I was included without knowing. We flew to Virginia. After a couple of days with Tia's friend, we rented a car and drove to Washington, DC. Sightseeing was educational, and the war memorials were emotionally moving. With a sea of names by the thousands, Arlington Cemetery made me feel unworthy to walk among such valor and honor. Endless crosses moved me to tears.

"God bless them," I said.

We arrived at a hotel aptly named Washington Hotel. Washington, DC, was like an antique picture someone tried to rejuvenate with cosmetics of paint and new fascia on fronts of old buildings in the older parts. I liked it. The nostalgic feel would outlast any attempts of re-coverings. There was a Chinese restaurant across the street from the hotel. The vertical storefronts accented the sidewalks that sloped down as if the road had dropped a few feet—I assumed because of the snow, to allow runoff, maybe. But it was very cold out, and if it did snow, there would be ice as well, and the sidewalk would be difficult to walk on. Well, it was Washington, DC, and more important things decided here made less sense.

We ordered Chinese food from the restaurant and returned to our room. For a hotel with the name Washington, you'd think the room would have been modest in its appearance, with drapes and bedcovers of an earth-toned color scheme. No, this room was purple all about and had a large clam-shaped Jacuzzi between the bedroom and the bathroom. Vegas! Or Hollywood, maybe.

How naïve of me, I thought.

We ate and took advantage of the Jacuzzi. It was a fun and educational trip in all.

18

Secret Admirers

Tia and I returned to work a few days later. Busy would be an understatement to describe some nights. You never stop moving. There's no real linear path for nursing. You prioritize. Constantly up and down the halls, I walked out of a patient's room and to the medication cart. In my absence someone left a toy-sized, gold-colored horse carriage full of chocolate candy kisses. A letter that accompanied it simply read, "From an admirer." This gift was not from Tia. As I was a resource nurse and worked all floors, I befriended doctors, nurses, and assistants. I looked up and down the hall. Everyone was in their own little worlds. No one looked up. I placed the candy in the nurses' station. I threw away the card. Candy and pastries of all kinds were a familiar sight in the nurses' stations of all floors. The chocolate candy kisses were eaten in time. I said nothing to Tia. A week later, after my shift ended at midnight, I walked out to my car, and the light from the building showed a word written in the dust that had collected on the trunk of my car. It read, "LOVE." I opened my car and took out a bottle of water from the cup holder. I washed the word and dust from the car trunk. The word remained scratched into the black paint—it was there to stay.

The next day at work, I mentioned what had happened among a few nurses and assistants at the station I worked the night before. I'd hoped word would get around, as it usually would, and further episodes could be avoided. This was not the case. Not two days had gone by, and as I opened my car door and sat down, I looked through my windshield. Several lipstick kisses blocked my view. I opened my trunk and retrieved a towel. My attempt to wipe off the lipstick did nothing but smear it. I pulled packets of alcohol wipes from my scrub top pocket, a normal accumulation of tools of the trade. This worked. I said nothing about this the following day. A week went by with no further incidents.

19

Do Not Crush

I walked into staffing like always to see what my assigned floor was.

"I need you over at the north campus to start tonight, William. I had a call-off, and I will try and get someone to come in to cover," Jenny from staffing stated.

This floor was the long-term care facility of the hospital, consisting of geriatric as well as head and spinal injuries. I had worked this floor before. I knew most of the nurses who called this long-term unit home. Rachel was a charge nurse whose talents were found primarily in her charting. Nice enough, Rachel was Italian; tall and slim; cute, in a word, with long, brown, braided hair that reached well past her waist. On her forehead was a decorative blue dot between her eyes, a common sight among women from India.

Odd. But to each his or her own, I thought.

When I walked in, Rachel looked up and smiled. "Are you here tonight?" she asked.

"Yes, but I don't know if it's all night. Jenny in staffing said she was working on someone to cover," I replied.

I took my patients report from the off going nurse and began the shift. An hour had passed with the routine duties of the floor, CNAs and nurses in and out of rooms attending to patients. Rachel stood up from her chair in the station. She walked into an adjacent break room behind the station. She reentered the station holding what appeared to be a towel. Rachel stepped out of the station and approached me at the medication cart.

"I have something for you," she said.

She presented me with a scrub top. The design was a copy of a sixteenth-century map of the world, gold and brown, with clipper ships and Chinese-looking dragons scattered about.

I thought, *Not one I'd wear while working pediatrics.*

Rachel said, "I bought it for myself, but I found it to be to masculine for me. I then thought of you."

Her brown eyes stared into mine. Rachel stood motionless as I looked at the top. Awkward, like a blind date unfolding in a nurses' station with coworkers looking on. I accepted it tactfully and thanked her for thinking of me. I wanted to know how long ago she purchased the scrub top.

Did she carry it with her? How did she know I'd be assigned to her floor? The thoughts culminated in my mind.

A few days had passed, and I was again assigned to work the long-term unit. Coming onto the floor, I greeted everyone in the vicinity like always. Making my rounds, I was approached by a certified nursing assistant (CNA), Gina, a young Mexican girl. She explained one of my patients wanted to speak to me. Mrs. Colwell, a morbidly obese woman of fifty years of age, lay in bed. Her medical history revealed that she had undergone a surgery some years prior in which both knees had been removed. Walking in, I observed another CNA assisting Mrs. Colwell. The assistant was holding an emesis basin.

"Mrs. Colwell was complaining of feeling nauseated and vomited twice," she said.

I went to the medication record to see if there was an order to give Mrs. Colwell something for nausea. There was: a 10 mg IM injection of Compazine, an antiemetic. As she was in fact throwing up, I held her one scheduled med at that time and wrote, per protocol, the reason on the reverse side of the medication administration record (MAR). A few days had passed, and I was assigned back on the long-term floor. Walking in, I was met by the charge nurse, Rachel, who gave me the scrub top days before. Only this time she had no smile for me. She rose from her chair with a shove that rolled it back three feet, and it stopped when it hit the wall. With one hand on a white ceiling support, she swung around it and approached me like I owed her money.

"Why didn't you give Mrs. Colwell her med three days ago?" she blurted abruptly.

Rachel's face was red, and she spoke with her teeth clenched. Two other nurses attempted to look busy, one at another medication cart and one at a treatment supply cart. Rachel stood aggressively glaring at me. I straightened in my stance and looked directly at her.

I asked, "Rachel, don't you think we should take this conversation to the nursing lounge?"

"I want to know! And right now," she retorted.

I then explained in detail my reason for holding Mrs. Colwell's med. I turned to the patient's medication page in the MAR.

I read my nurses' notes out loud. "Mrs. Colwell complained of nausea, and I observed emesis times two at this time. Compazine ten milligrams given intramuscular per doctor order. Will continue to monitor." A half hour later, per protocol, I wrote, "Patient still complaining of nausea with no further episodes of vomiting (emesis) at this time."

Rachel then belligerently and condescendingly said, "Why didn't you just crush it and put it through her G-tube?"

This is a gastric tube that goes directly into the stomach or the small intestines via a man-made stoma (a man-made hole in the abdomen for nutrition, water, and medications, which is accessible through a clear tube). Medications could be crushed and, with doctor-ordered increments of water should the patient be on a fluid restriction, administered through the tube with a 60 cc syringe.

I maintained my aura of naïveté. "Well, she does have a G-tube," I said like I hadn't thought of this route, for those in earshot.

I wanted all in attendance to think I had screwed up. I then asked the two other nurses, both of whom worked this floor and remained in the vicinity to watch the show unfold and had given Mrs. Colwell her medications prior.

"Is that what you do, Danny?, another L.V.N." I asked.

"And you, too?" I asked the other LVN standing at her medication cart opposite mine.

Both nurses said yes, as if to show they were in agreement with Rachel. Looking down at the medication sheet, I saw all their initials in giving medications on the days I wasn't there. I wanted to get them to verbally incriminate themselves, or, at the very least, show their incompetence as nurses. I turned to the MAR page that had the medication in question on it.

"Rachel, what does the SR90 stamped on the medication I held three days ago stand for?" I asked.

"That's not the point!" she snapped in reply, still very much glaring at me.

"No, I disagree. It is very much the point, and since you're the charge nurse for this floor, would you please educate those who obviously don't know?"

She just stood there at an obvious loss for words. I felt sorry for her. I had attempted to take this issue to the side privately and professionally, but Rachel wouldn't have it. I didn't take pleasure in my defense; OK, maybe I did enjoy the situation moderately. It was like having a royal flush during a poker game, as I knew now I would win this hand that publically questioned my level of medical competencies, and my character. It was my only option.

I then explained, "The SR stands for sustained release. The ninety stands for the milligram strength of the medication. The medication in question is morphine. With four days left in the month, I was the only one to hold this medication. Everyone else gave this medication, and by your own admission, you crushed it and administered it via the G-tube. It's also been made clear to me through the patient report that Mrs. Colwell has a psychiatric evaluation scheduled because she had been verbalizing that she drove her brother to Los Angeles as well as having participated in a running marathon. All this from a lady that five years earlier had both knees removed surgically. So I guess we can call off Dr. Stevens, the psychologist, now that we know the real reason for Mrs. Colwell's hallucinations, indicative of a morphine overdose. The medication SR90 morphine is con-traindicated that this medication should be crushed!" I finished.

Rachel turned and swiftly walked back behind the nurses' station and picked up a nurses' drug handbook. Pulling her chair back, she sat down and placed the book in her lap and flipped through the pages, pulling up the medication in question.

"Look down at the bottom of the page for three bold, italic words, 'Do not crush,'" I said.

Rachel sat and stared at the drug book's exoneration of me. The two other nurses waited in silence, still lingering at their carts. Rachel reached across the desktop that surrounded the inside of the nurses' station and picked up a black Sharpie marker and a yellow highlighter. She walked out of the station and to the medication cart. I took a step back. She wrote at the bottom of the medication sheet, "Do not crush," and then highlight-ed it with the yellow highlighter. Shutting the medication book, Rachel walked calmly back behind the station. Sitting back in her chair, she pulled a patient's chart she had in front of her and went about her task of chart-ing. Not a word. I was left standing by the medication cart. No apologies, nothing but silence. It was the cold shoulder again given by these nurses. I was now a social pariah because I advocated for a patient.

The patient had been given 90 mg of morphine bolus. What should have taken twelve hours to release the medication was given all at once. All three nurses didn't have a clue they were overdosing Mrs. Colwell.

I knew the real reason for Rachel's anger. I did not reciprocate her de-sired expectations of me for having given me a gift. Weeks earlier she had volunteered information about herself, that she went to India once a year to pray to an elephant; I believe it was an elephant. Maybe next time she could pray that the elephant could help with her memory of pharmacology.

With each night, I'd try and prepare for the inevitable and found my preparations were left wanting. I always thought it would be hard to adjust to the acute hospital. That maybe I'd make a poor showing in my abilities as a nurse. I realized I had nothing to worry about. The competition, if present, was sorely lacking.

20

Pediatric Pierced Nipple

The next week came, and I was approached by another charge nurse in pediatrics—Linda, another newcomer to the hospital. She was a young woman of approximately twenty-three, short in stature and maybe ten pounds overweight. She had a bubbly personality and was nice and approachable, a good quality for a nurse. The phone rang, and Linda answered it.

"Ped's [short for pediatrics]...He's right here." Linda said and handed me the phone.

"Hello, this is William."

The voice on the phone was Lisa, a nurse in ICU, asking me to come over and start an IV for them. "We've tried seven times, and the vein keeps blowing," she said.

I replied, "Sure, I'll try and will be right there."

I asked Linda, "Cover me?" Linda smiled and nodded. I walked to ICU.

I entered the unit, and all I needed to start an IV was placed on the counter below the telemetry monitors. Gathering the supplies, I went into the patient's room, a lady of maybe ninety years old with paper-thin skin. There were four-by-four gauzes taped across seven previously failed IV sites. I witnessed three-inch skin tears at two of them.

They had used tourniquets. When tied around the extremities, tourniquets pull the skin with the elasticity, and with a patient of this age, it tears his or her skin. And the pressure of blood that comes with a tourniquet blows the already-weakened vein. I abstained from making the same mistake and laid the patient's hand flat with the bed and unwrapped the IV supplies. The elderly patient was unconscious. Swabbing the patient's right hand, I picked out a blue vein and stuck the needle in bevel up. I pulled out the steel needle and pushed the plastic catheter's length all the way in. I taped the site and dated it. Hooking up the port to the saline bag already hung, I pushed start. I collected the remnants of the supplies, throwing them in the trash and the needle in the used-needle receptacle as I exited the room.

Lisa saw me enter the station and said, "Couldn't get it?"

I replied, "Yes, I got it. You're up and running at one hundred twenty-five drops a minute. Is that correct?"

Lisa answered, "Yes, and thank you, William."

I replied, "You're quite welcome"; washed my hands; and went back to pediatrics.

Linda was motoring about the station, looked up, and smiled. "You do it?"

"Yes, everything copacetic here?"

Linda replied, "Just fine."

Opening a chart to the doctors' order sheet, Linda turned the chart toward me. "I have to start an IV on Timothy," she said hesitantly.

Timothy was a four-year-old patient admitted for pneumonia. These were the worst for a nurse. At least they were for me. Little kids didn't understand the necessity for such invasive procedures.

I said, "I'll do it for you."

"Would you, William?" Linda replied.

"I'd do the same for an ICU nurse," I said, and smiled. Linda was young and new to nursing. I could tell she was uneasy or inexperienced with IVs.

"And, Linda, you better prepare yourself for future IVs and needle sticks," I said, stating the obvious.

Linda had verbally stated she always wanted to be a pediatric nurse, apparently not giving much thought to what that entailed. The evening went smoothly.

She asked, "What do you do after work for fun?"

"I usually go straight home, with an occasional stop at Judge Roy Bean's bar."

"By yourself?"

"No, I meet my friend Jerry usually."

"You meeting him tonight?" Linda queried.

"I haven't spoke to him as yet."

"Call him. We should go. My friend is meeting me after work tonight. I live in Ventura, and we don't know any place out here to go," she said.

I called Jerry, and again, Jerry was the younger brother of Ron, from my brief Ford automotive position, and explained the situation.

"Sure, I'll go," he replied.

I walked to the nurses' station to tell Linda the night was a go. The station was empty, and I assumed Linda was with a patient. I walked down the hall to a supply room, in need of a bag of saline to hang. I heard Linda's voice behind an adjacent door marked Nurses' Lounge. It was a one-sided conversation, broken up, pausing, in choppy words. Linda was on her cell phone encouraging a friend to drive out to Simi Valley. I quickly realized she hadn't made plans for the evening in the least. I walked back up the hall and into a patient's room where I changed out a near empty bag of saline for the new one. I checked the calculation for the drop ratio. I thought, *Better safe*, and pushed start.

Linda passed the door, and I walked out behind her. I said nothing of her private call moments earlier.

"Jerry says he'd be up for a nightcap at midnight," I said, signing off on my patient's input/output paper for the saline fluid.

Linda asked, "What kind of bar is it?" while pulling papers out from her white scrub top with smiling brown teddy bears in red and blue vests scattered all over.

"The kind of bar that serves alcohol," I replied in fun.

"I mean dancing, sports, you know."

"Yes, I know. A sports bar during the week. Both a sports and dance bar on the weekends, with a band."

I liked this bar. It had nice oak woodwork and booths, brass poles all about, dimly lit amber lights recessed into the ceiling, and an ambient 1920s speakeasy glow.

It was a welcome change from the hospital's florescent lights, which gave me headaches on occasion. I had been blessed with twenty-ten vision, and my eyes were a teal green that caught a lot of attention, as well as a lot of the florescent light I attributed to the headaches.

A jukebox sat in the division between the bar and two pool tables. Brighter lights hung over the billiard tables. I preferred to sit in the mellow-lit side of the bar and listen to music of an equally mellow nature on the jukebox, after work nights especially.

Standing in the nurses' station, Linda separated the papers in her hand. She singled one out.

"Here," she said, holding it out to me.

She handed me a photo. Other nurses had shown pictures here and there of family, babies, friends, and such. This photo she handed me with a smile and a matter-of-fact way was a clear, up-close view of her breast, to show me she'd just had a piercing through one of her nipples.

"Ouch!" is all I said, and handed it back.

"I was thinking of doing the other, too," Linda replied, looking down at the photo in her hand.

"I would consider removing the one you have," I said. Turning back to review the medication administration record for my patients.

"I have to check a blood sugar," I commented, and picked up a blood-sugar monitor and exited the station. The last few hours went routinely. Linda and I gave our patient reports to the oncoming nurses.

I strapped my stethoscope around my neck and grabbed my clipboard. As we both walked down the hall, Linda walked back in the nurses' lounge and retrieved a leather bag. She paused and opened it up. She pulled the papers and the photo from her scrub top and returned them to the bag. I looked down the dim-lit hall that appeared deserted with the approaching midnight hour.

"My friend is waiting in the parking lot," she said.

"Jerry said he'll meet us at the bar. Just follow me over."

Tia had been in Hollywood for a few days with family visiting from Manila, Philippines. Tia and I had an understanding: we were exclusive. Tia vaguely described me as "guys like you." I knew this night would get around the hospital, like some television soap opera. And I knew I would not have to worry about it, maybe. I trusted Tia, and she was going to have to do the same with me. Our convoy of two cars breeched the driveway of the large concrete corner lot from Cochran Street, east of Tapo Canyon Boulevard. A 7-Eleven on the left ended, and the beige walls of Judge Roy Bean's bar began.

We pulled in and parked. I saw Jerry's black Mustang parked a few rows over and felt relieved he showed. Linda's friend was quiet. Her name was Vanessa, a cute Mexican girl, about Linda's age, twenty-three, with long black hair and equally dark eyes. Vanessa was a kidney-dialysis nurse in Oxnard, California. Linda's flirtations of an obvious nature went interrupted by me with trips to the bathroom or to the jukebox for another song. I wasn't going to make the situation more than just friends out for a drink, so I kept my distance. I spoke more with Vanessa about work-related issues. Vanessa sipped her White Zinfandel, and I took a moderate swallow of my Jack Daniels and Coke to stave off a bit of anxiety. If I had not been involved with Tia, I would have pursued Vanessa, who seemed to be a sweet, intelligent, young woman. I would have only started with an invitation for a future outing with just us two. Linda had moved on to Jerry earlier, and for the most part, they got along famously. It was the second time this night Jerry's presence gave me a sigh of relief.

I usually would not date someone from work—this was too close to home, and, more important, work. Tia and I rarely crossed each other's paths at work.

The next day, I was off. Jerry called me in the afternoon.

I found out Linda had gone home with Jerry and spent the night. He'd just gotten home after driving Linda back to Ventura. I asked about

Vanessa. She and Linda followed Jerry to his house, and Vanessa drove home alone.

Two days had passed. The night with Linda had been brought up by a passing respiratory therapist (RT), Ronald, another player in the world of hospital characters. A past hospital encounter left Ronald's feelings hurt. His comments were an attempt to reciprocate in kind.

Ronald was a nice enough guy in general. He had short black hair and a short, blunt body, and he was heavyset with little to no neck to speak of. He was what many referred to when I was driving the emergency critical care team (CCT) ambulance in Los Angeles as a "Ricky Rescue."

He had a self-absorbed state of importance fueled by pretty lights and sirens. Only this was the hospital setting, not an intersection dividing the corners of four city blocks where bodies lay strewn across the pavement in swirls of blood and motor-oil trails. It was my experience that the ones who became more animated in an emergency were the ones less comfortable with their own abilities to perform the specific tasks for which they had been trained.

21

Time of Death

It had been months earlier when a patient on the north campus long-term floor coded.

Full arrest.

She died.

"Code blue one twenty-six, code blue one twenty-six, code blue one twenty-six." The monotone voice thronged out over the hospital intercom.

The patient, Mrs. Clary, was a ninety-six-year-old white female and very much emaciated. With the code-blue call came an instant movement change with all appropriate participants. The result was the same as that of an anthill when disturbed with a stick. The crash cart was mobilized. Respiratory responded by way of Ronald, the RT. Stethoscopes were thrown around necks, and all were to converge on room 126.

Others responding included two charge nurses, the patient's nurse, me, and two certified nursing assistants. I was the first to enter the room followed closely by a CNA, Espie. This CNA was the one bringing to our attention the patient's arrest. The patient's nurse, Denise, called in the code.

Espie said, "I was doing my rounds and found the patient had no vital signs."

Espie, an older Mexican woman, was a CNA in the truest sense.

She was a common sight on the long-term floor, a competent certified nursing assistant, an asset to the hospital in my professional opinion—an obvious one to any competent nurse who relied on her skills.

At first glance the woman appeared to have been admitted for cancer. I have observed many advanced-cancer patients in my medical travels, and she was a prime candidate. As she was not my patient, my assumptions were irrelevant.

"Let's get a full backboard under her," I said.

I lowered the head of the bed, laying Mrs. Clary flat on her back.

Espie moved in accordance, retrieving the full-length backboard from just across the hall in a supply closet filled with "H" and "E" tanks of oxygen (O2) and a couple of wheelchairs. I stood over the patient and, with my left hand, placed two fingers on the lateral right side of her neck, checking for a carotid pulse. The back of my right hand I held close to her mouth and nose to detect air movement, my eyes on her chest.

No pulse and no symmetrical chest expansion meant no breath.

I checked her pupils with a penlight for the record. Pupils were fixed and dilated. I knew death, and this was it. Body temperature was cool to the touch, and it was obvious that nothing warm in the form of blood had recently flowed beneath the epidermis (skin). I held the backboard and flattened it adjacent to Mrs. Clary's side.

"Pull her to your side, Espie" I said.

Espie put her hands across Mrs. Clary's body and rolled her from right to left toward herself. I could see signs of early lividity, a pooling of blood that settles with gravity after the heart stops pumping it. I slipped the backboard under Mrs. Clary and centered her body. Mrs. Clary's nurse—Denise, a white female of about thirty years old with shoulder-length, reddish, straight hair—stood to the side of the bed in observance. Having worked around her at times in the recent past, I surmised she had not been a nurse very long. Not incompetent, she just had a slower reflex in her execution of her duties. It's something that speeds up exponentially with time and experience.

I asked, "What's Mrs. Clary's code status, Denise?"

"I don't know!" she replied, immediately running to the nurse's station to check Mrs. Clary's chart. A do-not-resuscitate (DNR) order would have saved a lot of time and energy. Ronald, the RT, entered the room as Denise ran out. I had the stark-red crash cart standing by on the left side of the bed and to my right. On top of the crash cart sat an "ambu" bag, a clear plastic bag used for patient ventilations", ambu", short for ambulation.

Ronald exclaimed, "Give me the ambu bag!" in his excited state of animation, flailing his arms across Mrs. Clary's motionless body.

"Hey! Slow down, Ron. My floor, our patient, my show," I replied.

Denise came back in the room and calmly stated, "She's a no code."

A no code is otherwise known as a DNR.

"At 9:36 p.m.," I stated while looking down at my watch.

Denise looked at me and said, "What?"

"TOD, time of death."

Denise looked back down at Mrs. Clary's lifeless body, like reality had caught up with her.

"Right. Time of death," she said.

She seemed to take a mental note for future reference.

Ronald stood with a full anatomical feral expression, puffed out and round, like a tick ready to pop.

"DNR. Good thing we did not start CPR. Once we start, we cannot stop. And with it already set down as a legal document of Mrs. Clary's wish not to be revived, we'd all be in trouble," I explained.

Ronald turned, waddling toward the door, and scoffed in reply as he exited the room.

Cardio equals blood flow. Pulmonary equals air flow. Resuscitation equals to revive. I have used CPR more times than I can remember. No amount of CPR was going to help Mrs. Clary.

Denise and I left the two CNAs to perform their postmortem duties on the body of the late Mrs. Clary, and we walked back to the nurses' station. I pulled out Mrs. Clary's chart from the steel rack and set it down next to Denise, who sat motionless in one of five black nursing-station swivel chairs. She may have not been a nurse very long, but she sure had that "thousand-yard stare" mastered.

"You OK, Denise?" I asked.

"Yeah, you're fast. One, two, three, and it was done," she said, turning her stare toward the chart. It was the same expression she had when looking down at the late Mrs. Clary moments ago.

I replied, "I've had practice, that's all. You'll get it down."

Denise said, "I hope not. I mean, it's going to happen, I know. I just hope not again anytime soon."

I said, "Nature of the beast. When in Rome!"

"This is a hospital, William," she said as if not having caught my meaning.

"Geography, Denise, It's only geography, our job."

I leaned over from my perch on the counter and turned the chart toward me and opened it.

I said, "You going to call Mrs. Clary's doctor and next of kin to advise?" A kind of gentle verbal push in the right direction.

I flipped over a few pages to Mrs. Clary's admission sheet. She had been admitted for a total hip replacement at the age of ninety-six.

I thought, *Amazing. I would have never guessed that diagnosis ever.*

I sat down in my own black swivel chair and employed the rollers at the bottom and pushed myself to the right side of the station's counter, five feet over on Denise's right. I opened one of my patient's charts, pulled out a pen, and clicked it. Turning pages, Denise put her index finger on Mrs. Clary's personal-information page, picked up the phone, and tapped out a number. She paused and then sat up slightly at attention. "Hello, Doctor, this is Denise, the charge nurse for Mrs. Ethel Clary. I'm calling to inform you that she expired at nine thirty-six this evening. No, sir, not yet. Thank you, Doctor, and to you."

Denise hung the phone up and turned her head right, toward me.

"He asked if I called the family yet," she said.

I looked up from my notes and over at her and said, "I gathered." Smiling, I said, "Did he tell you to have a good night, too?"

"Yes, he did!" Denise said, somewhat surprised I knew.

"You wish him one back?"

"I did," she replied.

"Mmm." I smiled.

She asked, "You've done this many times, haven't you?"

I replied, "Yes, several. You'll get to the point, and soon. It's as easy as working a drive-through burger joint and asking if they want cheese on it."

I could see in her eyes that I had interpreted that she was having second thoughts about her occupational choice.

With more compassionate diction, due to the recent circumstance, I stated, "'We are what we repeatedly do. Excellence, then, is not an act, but a habit,' Aristotle said that."

Denise smiled back at me and then turned to the phone again and picked it up.

I went back to charting in my nurses notes.

The phone receiver lifted and *tap, tap, tap,* silence, and then, "Hello, Mr. Clary? This is Denise, the nurse for your mother. I'm sorry, sir, but Mrs. Clary passed away this evening at nine thirty-six in her sleep."

After a few more responses to the normal questions asked ("Did she suffer? Was she in pain at all?"), Denise said, "I'll call Reardon's Mortuary". A common destination for those of whom passed away, and was written down on Mrs. Clary's personal-information page. I'm sorry for your loss, sir. Good night."

Denise hung up the phone. I looked back toward her over the white counter reflecting the lights from the fluorescents overhead.

I said, "You're a natural, Denise. You're going to be fine."

Denise grinned and said, "I think I'm ready for med-surg or DOU [the direct observation unit]. Maybe the ER!"

I replied, "Where the action is! That's the spirit!"

Denise said, "Maybe in time. Tonight was action enough for a while."

I thought, *A professional night. An educational night. And Mrs. Clary's last night.*

As for Ronald, he never again stopped to speak amiably with me as he usually did in the past. We had "rank and filed" in the trenches, and he sulked as if he were a child disciplined for acting out. His comment about my night out at Judge Roy Bean's with Linda was his attempt at causing me emotional discomfort—Ronald's second failure in his abilities when it came to me.

22

Time, Money, and Manipulation

Tia confronted me in the hall between rehab and overflow. Tia stood with her arms crossed. "So I have to hear about this from others?" she said.

I replied, "You mean from Ronald?"

I could tell Tia was upset; the reason would have eluded me if not by the remark from Ronald about the night out with Linda and her friend. Ronald's attempt to unnerve me rolled away like water off a duck's back. No need to get flustered about something that did not exist. However, for Tia, it took up residence and jaded her.

Tia said, "He said—"

"*Stop!*" I stepped forward and lightly pulled Tia's arms apart. "I did nothing wrong. I'll not stand here and defend myself when there's nothing to defend. Get over your lingering adolescent high-school jealousies. Believe me, or believe Ronald. I went out after work, I had a couple of drinks, and I went home alone," I said.

Tia looked hard in my eyes for evidence of foul play on my part. The first of many stares, if I let it happen. I knew I would have to defend my life as long as she was a part of it. I turned and left Tia standing outside the station of physical rehabilitation and walked down the hall and went back to work in med-surg. Tia remained distant, like she was waiting for me to apologize. Since I had nothing to be sorry for, she had a long wait. I knew the poison of gossip worked its way into Tia's and my relationship. No trust meant no us. I had endured many of the same situations with past girlfriends and knew it was a losing battle. I saved myself the aggravation of the inevitable, long, drawn-out internal conflict to come and moved on. Better a quick death than the alternative, metaphorically speaking.

After nine or ten hours on a hospital floor, your feet and brain needed closure. I say nine or ten hours because any nurse will tell you, there is no such thing as an eight-hour shift. A new admission. A discharge. A transfer. A fall. A code. These all added another hour or two to your occupational plate. Sleep on many nights needed no nightcap of any kind. A dose of exhaustion put one flat on one's back. A few goings-over of the night's responsibilities in one's head, and the dream state of rapid eye movement (REM) replaced all the central nervous system's (CNS's) voluntary movements with the autonomic nervous system's (ANS's) forte of keeping the heart beating and air in the lungs. But there was change in the air, change in the hours.

I found I was getting called off at four hours into a shift. Sometimes whole shifts. I had been paid by the hour, and had two differentials. This meant more money per differential. One, if I worked seventy-two hours, or more, I'd be paid a few dollars more an hour. And if I worked my full weekend shifts, I was compensated again equally. The two differentials together were substantial in the scheme of things.

I was scheduled three to eleven and assigned to the direct observation unit (DOU). The DOU was a step-down unit from the intensive care unit (ICU). The unit always seemed darker, more shadowy than the rest of the floors of the hospital. It gave a feeling of working in a basement. With the other floors, they had large, open, protruding nurses' stations lit up in florescent lights that shone out onto the floors and down the halls. The DOU nurses' station was inset off the hallway that had a faded, but still dark, green fire door down the hall to the east. And to the west the hall ran straight into the med-surg floors past the brown solid-wood doors of the ICU. The hospital was forty or more years old. DOU had darker carpet and paint as well as equally dark-colored curtains that encircled patients' beds for privacy. Telemetry antennae hung from the ceilings in increments of thirty feet apart. And below them, walls of pale-blue wallpaper. A single door led into the nurses' station. The only two windows were maybe four feet square to the outside, and these were blocked by shrubs. The other window faced the dark hall, and a third of that was covered by books and racks of Xeroxed floor documents. There was one charge nurse, Carol, for the station. She was a rather full-figured white female of maybe forty-five years of age with strawberry-blond hair cut short in a bob. She manned the station while another nurse and I ran the floors. The other nurse, Maria, was a regular DOU floor nurse. She was Mexican with black hair pulled in a ponytail. She had fifteen patients. Over the past two years, my brown hair had grown out to shoulder length, and I had worn it in a ponytail as well, and I, too, had fifteen patients. The DOU was filled to capacity. Maria and I both worked manically about the unit. To the untrained eye, it was chaos, but to us it was multitasking at its best. It was a very busy night, in and out of the station for doctors' orders, charting nurses' notes, intravenous (IV) supplies, and intramuscular (IM) and by-mouth (PO) pain medications. I briskly entered the station. Carol was on one phone, and another line rang. I stopped and picked it up.

"DOU, this is William."

The call came in from admitting. "We have one coming in to be admitted to your floor," the nameless voice declared.

I replied, "Are you aware we are maxed out of beds on this floor?"

Carol finished her call and hung up and then turned her attention to me.

The voice said, "You'll have to put the patient in the hall."

"Put the patient in the hall?" I exclaimed in a surprised tone but more as a warning to Carol. I turned to her.

She was squeezed into her chair. She had rolled back a foot and stared up at me while listening to the one-sided conversation.

I asked the voice, "How long till the patient arrives?"

The voice replied, "One hour. We'll call back then." And the phone went silent.

"They're admitting another patient to us in one hour," I said to Carol.

"No, they're not," she replied, and swung her chair back into the center of the station's counter and picked up the phone. I exited the station and continued with the duties of the floor. An hour came and went. With some juggling of patients, two were moved to med-surg, our admission was accommodated. No break tonight for anyone.

With staffing calling me off, I started my own investigation of time cards and corresponding days. It got to the point where I could call it to the hour. This was the case in DOU. I entered the station. Maria was charting in her notes and Carol was writing in the new admission's chart.

"Carol, it's five minutes to seven, and I'm getting called off," I stated.

Turning suddenly in her chair toward me, she asked despairingly, "Are you sick?"

Maria stopped writing and looked across the station at me then Carol. "No, I'm fine," I replied.

Carol asked, "Why, then? You can't leave us like this!"

"I wouldn't, Carol, but I have no choice," I said. "Within another three minutes, the phone will ring, and it will be Jenny from staffing."

Carol stared at me in silence, and Maria stood motionless to my left with a look of panic in her watery dark eyes. Just then the phone rang. All three heads turned in sync to the direction of the sound. They looked back at me in disbelief. I shrugged and gestured with my hand toward the phone that continued to ring. Carol broke from her shocked stare and pushed and swiveled her chair all at the same time across the laminate-tile floor and toward the counter.

Snatching the phone off its cradle and placing it to her ear, she said, "DOU, Carol!" She paused in the silence.

Carol said, "Yes, William's standing right here. He was just telling us that."

She held the phone in her left hand and placed her right elbow on the counter. Carol put her forehead in her right hand like she was checking for a fever and shook it back and forth slowly.

"We are so busy tonight; we're full here," she said, distraught.

Looking back at me from her cradled lolling head, Carol handed me the phone with an outstretched left arm. Her right elbow was still attached to the counter.

"Hello, Jenny."

"Yes, good evening, William. We're calling you off at seven," Jenny replied in a matter-of-fact tone.

I said, "What if I punch out and remain the last four hours. We're swamped in here."

Jenny replied, "No, insurance wouldn't allow for that."

"No way then?" I asked.

"No, at seven you're off the clock. Good night, Will."

I hung the phone up.

Carol asked, "How did you know they were going to call you off?"

Maria walked over to the counter and leaned against it with her own look of curiosity.

"Well, I have worked sixty-eight hours as of tonight. I, like many others you know, get paid a differential for working seventy-two hours in a two-week pay period. I also get paid a differential for not missing any days or hours during my scheduled weekends. At sixty-eight hours and this being a Sunday, the hospital calls me off, nullifying both differentials."

Carol said, "And saving a chunk of money."

"If I finished the last four hours of this night, it would be the opposite," I replied.

Maria responded, "And we have to suffer?"

I nodded my head. "I'm afraid so. Carol; you; me; and, most important, the patients. I'm sorry."

Carol said, "It's not your fault!"

I gave the report to Maria on my patients and picked up my stethoscope. Patients' call lights with their accompanying buzzers sounded, all for Maria's attention now. I turned and exited the DOU.

23

Methadone Clinic

The dark DOU halls faded as light from other stations engulfed me. My thoughts turned to a methadone clinic, one of three in particular. This one was located in Van Nuys, California. I was hired to fill the one and only nursing position, with the sole purpose of dispensing methadone. It was an equally dark and dismal facility that mirrored the DOU. I had my own office where no one was allowed, not even the facility's manager. There were copious amounts of DEA-controlled methadone locked in a safe, and I was the only one with the combination and license to access it. Almost all the counselors—four Hispanic females—were ex-heroin users. The manager told me she hadn't been a user. Most had tattoos about their bodies and necks, gang insignias and names of people that are, or were, in their lives.

At four in the morning, I'd arrive and unlock the back door that faced an alley. I made sure of my surroundings as this particular part of town and, of course, the nature of this facility behooved one to be on guard. I would shut off the alarm and turn on the lights. The facility was poorly lit. A dingy, dark-green carpet was matted down from years of traffic of the afflicted. The walls at one time had been white but now were faded dull with scuffs and moderate amounts of graffiti. The door that faced the alley opened to a long hallway that ended in a waiting room of dark-brown paneling with approximately twenty chairs of plastic and steel. It was a square, like in most medical offices, with a long counter that divided that room from the manager's office and mine. Patients would arrive starting at five and give their names if new, but for the most part, the receptionist would give a nod of recognition, pull the patient's card with his or her picture on it, date it, and bring to my office. I would place them in the order I received them and dose accordingly.

My door was, of course, a full door but cut in the middle, which allowed the bottom to be kept locked while dispensing. On top of the door's bottom half was a small, white platform. The first day, this foot-wide platform was dirty with fingerprints and general smudges of spilled drops of the liquid methadone mixed with the dirt of hands and a few patients' articles of clothing, for they called the alley and streets home. I recall this was the first thing I washed, leaving it a bright white. My office, having far less traffic, was fairly clean and had two rectangular tables and a large safe in it. The walls were brown paneling. After a few days, I had brought in, at my own expense, some higher-watt florescent bulbs, cleanser, and a few air fresheners. I found a vacuum buried under some boxes of paper towels and cups used to mix the individual amounts of doctor-ordered methadone. I employed this vacuum every day after the shift ended, which was at one in the afternoon. I brought a colored landscape picture of a lake and trees, about four feet square and encased in a gold frame, that dominated the wall behind me as I faced patients. I could tell after a week that the general mood of those who dosed there had improved greatly.

Now most would probably think of heroin users as homeless alley dwellers—I know I used to—but I soon found that approximately 80 percent were your average neighbor types. People on their way to work, in all occupations.

About two weeks had passed. Laurie, the LVN I was replacing, was heading up to Carson City, Nevada. Laurie had decided to move there, hence the open LVN position.

"William? Can you cover this weekend for me?" Laurie asked.

"Sure, I can do that. You're covered," I replied.

The week came and went, as did that weekend. Since the next weekend was mine to cover per the regular schedule, I worked sixteen days in a row.

When Laurie was to be back the following Monday, my day off, she called in sick, and, subsequently, I was called in to cover. Day seventeen.

Laurie was a professional in all aspects of being a nurse. She shared my approach toward our responsibilities. Her personal life was characteristic of a twenty-three-year-old. There were parties. There were modifications done to her Honda Civic: lowered and custom rims, tinted windows, and an impressive sound system.

Laurie's trips up to Carson City, Nevada, became more frequent, and her departure felt imminent. Another week had passed uneventfully.

At four in the morning, I started the day's routine. I opened my office and set up. The hall to the back where my office and the manager's were located was an L shape. The manager's door was just to the right from mine, and her desk, where she sat most of the day, was no more than ten feet away. I could, and often did, ask Gina a question, and she me with little effort in hearing one another. Gina was Mexican and nice to work with. She had two children and had been married happily for the past five years. I can say "happily" because of the many visits from her husband, Jessie. He'd bring Gina her lunch, and they'd eat together, talking and laughing. Never a bad comment or degree of a fight. No forced pleasantries. I could say they weren't only married, they were friends. I admired them for this. And as I said, I could easily hear from my office door. Laurie, however, had been distant, in thought really more than anything. Her wheels were turning in her mind about something. I never felt absolute in believing Laurie was 100 percent on leaving and moving to Carson City. Laurie's enthusiasm about this endeavor had tapered off, and I noticed. Nothing was said, but it was in the air.

This particular day, I was setting a CD in the small stereo I'd brought in with the landscape picture that hung on the wall. I'd play CD's of Enigma or *Pure Moods*, just a soft instrumental backdrop, like elevator music, to break the morose silences.

"William, may I speak with you for a moment please?" Gina asked from her seat behind her desk.

"On my way," I replied.

I walked into her office and stood in front of the desk.

"Good morning, Gina," I said with a smile.

It was four forty-five, and some of the patients had strolled in and were waiting in the waiting room down the hall. I had a camera that showed the whole front of the clinic and an intercom used to call back each patient one at a time.

"William, I've had some complaints about you," she said.

"Oh? And they are?" I replied. My smile went on break to leave us alone.

"Well, a few people said you smelled of alcohol. Vodka was named."

"So I'm cruising down the 405 at three thirty in the morning, coming in to work and guzzling down a bottle of Grandpa's O'l- cough medicine?" I said, my defenses growing. "What else?" I asked.

"That you've been making improper sexual comments to the female patients when they come in to dose," Gina continued.

"My only contact with any of these patients happens right outside my office door, ten feet from you. I am the nurse. I have access to all patients' charts and information. At the very least, a third of these patients have hepatitis; a few have HIV. I could be in a club, or a library, it doesn't matter! I'd never conduct myself in such a vulgar manner," I stated sternly.

Gina continued as if building grounds for my immediate dismissal from my position.

"Another patient claimed you solicited him for some heroin," she said.

"*What!* You think I'd go through one of these mental giants to score some smack? And that I'd eagerly wish to join their ranks?" I retorted.

"*No!* No, I don't believe that you did," she said.

"Which part? This is a fucking witch-hunt, this is! You're not sharing with me patient issues; you're accusing me straight up!"

Then the lack of Laurie's enthusiasm, and now this made sense to me.

"Laurie's no longer moving to Carson City; therefore, there's no longer a need for two nurses!" I stated.

"Oh! So she spoke with you?" Gina asked.

Her question justified my hunch. "No! I'm not stupid! But instead of just telling me the truth up front, you apparently felt the need for my vilification as a drunk, womanizing, fledgling heroin user! If you'd given me the simple truth, I'd have wished you all the best and thanked you for the opportunity, and we would have parted ways as friends," I vented profusely.

I continued. "You'd have fared better to have held court on me after one o'clock, after all the patients had taken their dose.

Fuck this! And fuck you."

"Do you want to watch your language?" Gina said.

"My language? Every other word from any of you here is 'fuck,' so fuck you. Fuck you twice!"

I walked out of Gina's office and into mine. I unplugged the stereo and grabbed a small plant and humped it to my car out back. I came back in and claimed my picture from the wall and repeated the trip.

"Are you leaving?" Gina asked.

"Figured that out, did you?" I sarcastically answered her.

"Wh-wh-what?" Gina stuttered.

"Laurie lives two minutes from here—call her in," I stated.

"She called in sick, and—"

"I know! I took the call. 'Hangover' was the reason she gave me. Tell her to take a shot or two of the hair of the dog, spike a vein, and come in to work!" I retorted.

I was furious with having to contend, time after time, with the confrontational, lying, condescending thrusts of the tongue that seemed to follow me from place to place, like I was playing a flute and leading a company of rats. I stayed and dosed a dozen patients waiting for Laurie's arrival. She came in, and I left.

The practice of my patience was losing ground.

24

Single Again

I attended picnics, parties, and Bar Mitzvahs with many of my coworkers, male and female. It's called life; and I came to play.

Jerry and I accompanied Connie, a nurse, and another platonic friend of the florescent floors of the hospital, and her friend Laura, both from Moorpark, California, to a night's excursion out to unwind. From past experience, going out with coworkers proved to be detrimental. I wasn't worried though. I only had myself to answer to. And when driving an ambulance, we were told we'd spend more time with our partners than with any wife or girlfriend we had. I found this to be true. This is the reason most are involved with people of the same occupation, or closely related in some way to it. Lawyers date lawyers. Doctors, nurses with the same. Bull fighters, I don't know about. I suggested going to Hollywood, to a club I was familiar with. The Monkey Bar on Melrose. A club that if you didn't know it was there, you'd drive right by. The Monkey Bar was covered in ivy.

The roof and exterior walls were nothing but green ivy. We arrived early enough to get a booth, or it was just timing. A band played from the southeast corner of the club to a packed house. There was no bandstand to speak of. "Mustang Sally" was the song. The lead guitarist walked on the flat, six-inch-wide beige banister that divided the tables, ducking down so he wouldn't hit his head on the overhanging brass lights. As in the movie-production world of Hollywood, it's taboo to bother the actors or musicians. The Monkey Bar had a mixed crowd of both well-known people—Hollywood stars or celebrities, if you will—and not so well-known people. I fell in the latter category. This was a bar where the well-known could just be. This was a club not found on any maps of Hollywood. Tourists were not privy to the knowledge of such an exclusive haven. I explained this to Jerry, who for the most part rarely got out of Simi Valley. When we arrived at the bar, there were about fifty paparazzi snapping pictures. It was like a lightning storm on crack. The night was very exciting. There were no hidden agendas from Connie or Laura. None from Jerry or me. Having a modest number of drinks in me, I was glad that Connie's friend Laura was driving. She had maybe two drinks earlier in the night and then switched to 7 Up. Laura was a little high strung for the Hollywood crowd. She had stated she felt out of place, and it showed.

About midnight we all walked out of the Monkey Bar and proceeded up the street to Laura's car. I could see a familiar sight of a stage-light glow coming out elongated, rectangular windows on the front of a building. I walked over and looked through the windows in curiosity. It was a photo shoot with the actress and model Grace Slick posing glamorously for the camera. We all continued walking up the sidewalk, a successful feeling of accomplishment in that it was a good night, our objective. Comments made by Jerry confirmed this feeling, when he expressed his amazement with the whole night. "Star struck" is the term. We drove north on Highland Boulevard through the streets of Hollywood, past the Hollywood Bowl and onto the 101 freeway north. They dropped me and Jerry off at my apartment. Connie and Laura politely thanked us for our company and the night in general and calmly drove off.

I thought, *The way a night should go. No anger because one failed to read between the lines of another's presumptuous expectations. No drama.*

25

Two O'clock A.M. Retaliation

Back to the routine of work, home, relatives, movies, concerts, surfing. Maybe a week had gone by since the Hollywood excursion. The end of a late-night shift, I left work tired and drained—a great feeling really—went straight home, and undressed. I showered and went to bed. It was two in the morning when my phone rang. A strident demand for attention. Depending on what side of my California king-sized bed I was on, I reached for one or the other phone I had on either side. I thought maybe a family emergency, or just a wrong number. Or someone was sick and needed coverage at work.

"Hello, this is William," I said, still with my eyes closed.

"Hello, William? Do you want some company?" said a slurred but familiar voice. It was Connie, the nurse from work, and last week's Hollywood outing. I knew she was married and had kids. I wanted no part of this. My first instinct was to verbally back off like a spider on a hot stove, but knew I'd better, at least for the moment, make a window for her to save face. I knew she had been drinking by her slurred speech.

"Connie, you shouldn't be driving a wheelchair let alone a car," I lightly said.

"Whatever!" she shouted and abruptly hung up. Not the outcome I strived for. At two in the morning and still half asleep from exhaustion, my usual wit was equal to the green, numbered lights from the now-silent phone still in my hand: dim. I hoped that maybe she wouldn't remember the call the next day. If she did, maybe not so much who it was she called. And maybe there was finally going to be world peace. These hopes were all in vain.

The next morning I went through my activities of daily living (ADL) routine. I showered and donned a scrub top and a pair of white 501 Levi's. I swung my stethoscope around my neck and clipped a couple of pens and my ID badge on my scrub pocket. My usual uniform. I drove west down Los Angeles Avenue and made a right, north on Sycamore Drive. I coasted around the hospital's parking lot and sank into a parking spot reserved for doctors only. Most of the doctors knew me, and I them, and no one ever complained. It was a nice day, and I was feeling content.

I thought, *Last night's two o'clock nightmare was a lifetime ago—no worries.* I walked in the front door of the hospital and into staffing.

I said, "Good morning, Jenny," to a stocky, short-haired blonde who sat snug in her chair against a desk of telephones and computer screens.

"Good day, Will," she said in reply, without looking up, peering stolidly through her glasses at the blinking lights.

Must get awfully lonely in her drab little office, I thought.

I turned to the office door with its faded brown stain with little holes sporadically about halfway up the door from past scheduling, including the day's three white schedule papers tacked in place. I looked to see what floor I was assigned: med-surg overflow. Then I looked to the left on the schedule for one of the numerous charge nurse's names. Connie! My late-night caller.

I thought, *Damn! What'd I do? Lose a bet?* Thoughts of Jenny's isolation only moments ago seemed a bit more appealing.

Leaving the staffing office, I turned left and down the hall of the main hospital, out the exit and north down the sidewalk, and across the street. I walked through the north-campus door. It was quieter here than on the main floors of the hospital, probably due to the many administrative offices. Passing infection control, I entered the overflow unit and greeted a couple of certified nursing assistants and Connie. The assistants replied in kind. Connie did not.

Connie was a frail woman in appearance; slim; and short in height and in hair, which was dirty dishwater in color and unkempt.

I thought, *Too young to look that old.*

She was a completely different person from the night out in Hollywood a week before. Connie sat in a charcoal-colored padded swivel chair, inert behind the counter of the nurses' station. Hands and arms listless at her sides. A blank look. Dormant. If there was a winter season for the human being, Connie was in the dead of it. Neither of us said anything outside of issues relating to work. Even so, her voice was bland of any discernible tone as we quietly passed in the halls on occasion, going about performing our jobs.

Time clicked by uneventfully.

Connie was on the phone in the station. She wrote on a pad of paper. I turned my back to her and visually scanned timed medications on the medication administration record (MAR).

"OK, thank you, Steve," I heard Connie say, and the phone clacked in its cradle. I thought nothing of this, but I was also relieved to hear her speak in a calm and cordial tone.

I thought, *Maybe she blew off the late-night rejection from me and moved forward.*

An hour had passed, and Steve from pharmacy strolled down the hall and into the nurses' station with a bag of medications. Steve was a lanky guy, about six feet four, three inches taller than me. He had short brown hair that looked as if he cut it himself, it was so lopsided. Steve set the bag on the counter in front of Connie and leaned slightly down.

"Here ya go, Connie," Steve said in a drawn-out southern way.

Smiling up from her seated position, Connie replied, "Thank you, sweetheart."

Going about my duties, I walked past the station, leaving Connie, Steve, and the rustling sound of the pharmacy bag behind me. I checked on patients, hung a new bag of saline, and passed a few medications.

All was fine as clockwork. Back at the MAR, I signed off the meds I'd just given. I handed a piece of paper to a CNA with the increment of fluid from the bag of saline written on it.

I directed her. "Chart this in one eleven B's I and O, please."

The assistant smiled flirtatiously. I turned and came face to face with Connie. She appeared to have received good news, or just a moment of clarity; I'd take either one.

Smiling, Connie said, "I spoke with Dr. Leeds, for patient Mrs. Kane, and she's to start this medication, starting now and then once daily in the mornings."

I thought, *Amiable enough—no overtones of a negative nature.*

I held out my hand. "OK," I replied.

Taking the paper medication cup from Connie's hand with the medication already in it, I glanced at the single pill and recognized it. I turned from Connie and exited out of the station. I knew now what Steve had delivered from the hospital pharmacy. I walked south toward the patient's room. Connie kept pace six feet behind me. I gave her the benefit of *my* doubt that she wasn't following me and was merely going to another patient's room. I turned when we both passed the last door in the east hall leading to the specified room on the far south wing.

I asked, "Do you want to give this medication, Connie?"

She had stopped when I did. Defiant in her stance and face.

"No, you give it!" she retorted.

I walked the rest of the length of the hall, now knowing full well she was going to stand over my shoulder. This would never have happened except for the audacious two o'clock phone call. The old adage, "Hell has no fury like a woman scorned," came to mind. This was retaliation, an obvious ploy to get back at me from last night's refusal of her company. Connie's only hand to play was that she was the charge nurse for the floor. Charge nurses will occasionally delegate duties to other nurses of lesser ranks—an occasional, "Cover me," or "Start an IV." Only this time, it was done lacking tact.

I continued toward Mrs. Kane's room with Connie in tow.

I thought, *God, please let there be a family member at the bedside.*

As with my experience, the question you can and should always expect when giving a drug was, "What is it?"

And today it was very much in demand for my needs. I entered Mrs. Kane's room with a knock and a pause. Mrs. Kane lay in bed in a semi-Fowler's position, pleasantly smiling. At the foot of the bed was a woman of about fifty, who was heavyset with black hair and glasses with large, round, tinted lenses. It was Mrs. Kane's daughter. Mrs. Kane was about eighty years old. Late-afternoon sunlight shone warmly through the window.

I approached and greeted her. "Nice day, don't you think, Mrs. Kane?"

"Yes. Too fine to be indoors," she replied.

She was a nice woman, bright and cognizant.

"This is my daughter, Kate" she said proudly.

"Hello, Kate, my name is William."

"Nice to meet you," she replied placidly.

I explained to Mrs. Kane what the reason was for this specific visit. A tray with a cup and drinking water sat on Mrs. Kane's bedside table. I tipped the cup upright and pulled the top off the green plastic water container. I poured the cup halfway with the water.

"I have a new medication Dr. Leeds has ordered for you," I said, goading a response from either Mrs. Kane or her daughter.

Timing was everything. One prayer for the family member bedside answered; I prayed again for the inevitable question. Waiting, waiting, and—

"What is it?" the patient's daughter, Kate, asked.

I smiled and turned to where Connie stood, just inside the doorway with her arms crossed tight against her chest, still authoritatively aloof and dogmatic in her endeavor to make me compensate for her self-induced ignominy. I gestured toward Connie with my hand, putting Mrs. Kane's, and her daughter Kate's, attention on her.

I said, "Well, as you may know, Connie here is the charge nurse for this floor and spoke directly with Dr. Leeds. It was Connie who took the medication order and pulled the medication for your mother. She can best explain what the medication is and what it's for."

The whole time I was staring straight at Connie. With her bellicose demeanor changing, Connie's arms were uncrossing slowly and falling in a confused manner, down a bit, back up. Absolute loss of composure, her lips opened now from the previous thin-lipped grimace. She stammered in speech to start. Connie began to explain, like a politician who said everything and nothing, making no sense.

Realizing she was faltering, she said, "Because of all the medications of a cardiac nature, I will go look it up."

Connie turned slightly to exit. Opportunity raised its head, and I was going to exploit it. I couldn't have wanted it better. I had to show I wasn't going to be intimidated because I didn't want to sleep with Connie, if that was my choice. She was married. She had kids. I chose not to.

I spoke up. "That won't be necessary."

Connie stopped and stared blankly at the doorjamb, as if having no will to move forward or back, offering only a celestial gaze.

I turned to Mrs. Kane and picked up the paper cup holding the medication and said, "This medication decreases the preload and after-load of blood volume in the left ventricle of the heart. By decreasing the amount of fluid, it lessens the workload of the heart and, in turn, decreases the oxygen demand of the heart in its efforts to pump the blood through the aorta and back out through the body."

There was silence in the room for a couple of heartbeats.

Mrs. Kane said, "Well, that sounds good."

Kate said, "Yes, it does. Thank you."

I handed the medication to Mrs. Kane, and she poured it in her mouth.

A drink of water, and she swallowed it. With no further questions from the patient or her daughter, I left them to their visit, both smiling. I headed back to the nurses' station to sign off on the MAR. First, I was going to have to write the new medication down, something I was sure Connie had not done.

Connie briskly walked down the hall, ten feet in front of me now, and was hell-bent for the nurses' station. She sat abruptly in the swivel chair and snatched up a nurses' drug book like she was swatting a fly off a picnic table. She began flipping pages in what appeared to be a hysterical state. With her index finger pressed to the print, she reached the medication.

Her red face softened and began to pale to normal slowly. Her eyes glazed over a little as if she were going to cry. I took a step toward her.

Connie looked up at me and said, "That's word for word."

I replied, "Yes, Connie, I got an A in pharmacology. I endeavor to get As in everything."

Truth is, I look up medications constantly. This drug, among many others, is commonly utilized, and one I was familiar with. My surprise was that Connie wasn't. The comment was a final gesture on my part to back her off. Connie just lobbed the drug book onto the white counter of the station and sank in her chair. The chair sighed with a squeak under Connie's weight. She appeared exhausted, physically and mentally. I turned and went about writing down the medication in the MAR. I felt a sense of remorse. Something in her manner, in general, told me that I wasn't the only demon she had to contend with. Her verbalized desires the night before may have been a last-ditch effort to feel alive. Maybe home life had reached an exhausting point. A stale routine of work and kids—an unappreciative, inattentive husband, maybe. Connie looked like the last of her spirit had run out. I worked quietly and remained calm and kind when work dictated that Connie and I had to converse. The rest of the night I went unopposed. We all just did what was expected of us to the best of our abilities. I'd rather this edifying medication event been discussed in a better professional arena, and may have been, if not for the two o'clock phone call. The night, the patient, and the medication still would have manifested. It was the animosities Connie held for me we both could have done without. As with doctors we, too, as nurses consult with one another. I recommend this highly as an educational tool. *No one* knows everything, especially with the new and constant augmentation of medications and procedures. It helps in communication skills and provides an all-around good feeling of being part of a positive, productive team. There's nothing wrong with asking a question, and it's equally less wrong in giving an answer. Second-guess only late-night phone calls.

26

Reducing Risk of UTI

Another long-term care, med-surg overflow floor shift. I tensed up when I was required to cover this floor where I was given the scrub top and gave the lecture on not crushing sustained medications. I got a cold-shoulder feeling from the usual nurses that ran this unit. Having already spent four hours on med-surg, I was called and sent to the long-term floor for the last four hours. I didn't know I was going there, and so never thought to look at the name on the schedule in staffing to see what charge nurse was on. Stepping across the foyer, I was relieved to see that it was a different charge nurse. New to the hospital, Riva was a young, attractive Filipino girl of about twenty-four years of age. She sat quietly behind the nurses' station, which I readily observed as awkwardness, a feeling of being new and out of place.

A new hospital, maybe her first. New people: me.

I had been on and off this floor about three times this week and was aware of the new patients and their individual diagnoses. Some of the patients were admitted first to the main med-surg floor, my home base, and then transferred to specialized floors. I was the admitting nurse for Mrs. Kindle when she was first admitted to med-surg. She had come into Simi Valley for her grandson's graduation. She had suffered a cerebral-vascular accident (CVA), a stroke. With two hemispheres in the brain, the infarction, or death of tissue in the brain, occurred on her left hemisphere, leaving the right side paralyzed. A crossing over, left to right, right to left, causing total loss of her right-side extremities and speech. Mrs. Kindle's mouth drooped down hard on the right side. She was absolutely helpless.

I recall a male patient, Mr. Anderson, many months earlier who was admitted for the same diagnosis of CVA. With anticoagulant medications, like Coumadin, and physical therapy, he was able to walk out of the hospital. I remember thinking what he suffered was probably a transient ischemic attack, (TIA), where a clot gets stuck long enough to restrict oxygenated blood flow to parts of the brain, an almost complete occlusion of an artery, causing temporary paralysis with no infarction (death) of tissue. It was maybe two months later when I saw him again. He was walking into the rehabilitation department to visit his wife, who had been admitted for a hip replacement.

Mr. Anderson was wearing golfing attire and just finished eighteen holes.

With Mrs. Kindle, it was a CVA, and she was going to be our guest for some time. I had already been made aware that a pending order for Mrs. Kindle still needed to be realized. The norm was for the doctor to call the order in. This night, the norm was out, and the doctor was in.

Dr. Moore, a urologist, walked in with an obvious mission. He was a stout man of about fifty-five, bald, with gray patches of hair just above his ears. He wore a yellow casual dress shirt and faded blue jeans. It looked as if he just got off a couch. He walked into the station, dominating space with his presence, and abruptly sat down. He swiveled the chair around, squelching and creaking to the steel-rack collection of patient charts, and grabbed Mrs. Kindle's. He tossed the chart from a foot away, and it landed with a slap on the counter.

Positioning himself, Dr. Moore blurted out, "Why am I here?"

He sat leaning and facing right toward Riva, not three feet away. This petite, pretty Filipino girl with shiny black hair that fell straight down to her lower back, with the sides pinned over her ears, sat like a rabbit that found itself in close proximity to a predator that saw her as its next meal. And if she didn't move, it would go away. Sheer fright in her eyes as she looked straight ahead with Dr. Moore looking straight at her. She had absolutely vapor locked. I was standing at the medication cart on the outside of the nurses' station, looking down diagonally at what was not going to be a pretty exchange of the doctor's verbal frustrations. Riva's right hand crept toward the seventy-two-hour patient-report sheet, a three-day collection of falls, infections, and impending doctors' orders. I knew what Riva looked for wasn't there.

I leaned on the medication cart and cleared my throat.

I said, "Oh, yes, Dr. Moore, I just changed over here from med-surg, and I was given the report by the off going nurse but have yet to speak with Riva here. And I apologize for the delay, Riva."

Dr. Moore looked up at me over Riva, who remained inert.

"You're here, Doctor, because we have been straight catheterizing Mrs. Kindle every eight hours for urine. She, as you may know, was admitted for a cerebral vascular accident, a stroke. And we needed you to tell us if you want us to continue with the straight catheterizing, or to apply an indwelling catheter and decrease the risk of a urinary tract infection, as she may be with us for a while."

Dr. Moore tapped his pen three times in thought. Turning back to the chart, he opened it to the doctor's order sheet.

"All right! Let's go with the indwelling catheter and change it once a month or as needed for plugging." He spoke as he wrote the order verbatim.

"Is that all you need from me?" he asked.

I replied, "Yes, sir, to my knowledge."

"OK, then." He closed the chart and lightly got up. Strolling out of the nurses' station, he said, "Have a good night."

"And to you as well, Dr. Moore. Thank you," I replied.

I looked back toward Riva, who was stolid, petrified in appearance. She still had not moved, and I wasn't sure if she was breathing. I had noticed all too frequently other nurses freezing up when speaking with doctors.

I then said, "Riva, I'm sorry if I overstepped my bounds."

Riva began to show signs of life by blinking her dark eyes.

"No! Not at all. I didn't know what to say. I received the patient report, but nothing was said of this. If you know something I don't, go right ahead," she replied.

I was sure she didn't mind by her sincere statement, a sigh of relief, and color returning to her face. Why this information was not communicated to her in the report by the charge nurse Riva took over for eludes me; however, the degree of importance of such information does not.

27

Death by Drowning

It would be a few days later that Darlene (another attractive Filipino girl whom I had met about a month prior in the med-surg overflow) and I would be covering this long-term floor.

Darlene was a sweet girl with a whimsical disposition. One might go as far as to say she was an "airhead." Much more a term of endearment than a condescending criticism. She was very enthusiastic and congenial.

Darlene, an RN, was the charge nurse, and she had received a lab showing a low level of potassium (K) for Mrs. Kindle, the patient from days before with the CVA stroke for which the indwelling catheter order had been written. Darlene called and made the primary doctor for Mrs. Kindle aware of this deficit of potassium.

Darlene received an order to add 10 mg of potassium (K) to a bag of normal saline and infuse it into the patient's IV heparin-lock port and run the medication in total over a period of one hour. Mrs. Kindle had a heparin lock, an access port for intravenous fluids, on her left arm. This was mostly to receive medications of one- to two-milliliter (ml) pushes. I have on many occasions had the same order for the same reason. I always added the potassium (K) myself. Draw up the doctor-ordered increment of liquid K with a twenty-three-gauge needle already connected to its plunger and push it into the saline bag's port. Shake the bag a little and hang it.

Instead of Darlene mixing it herself, she called on the hospital's pharmacy to do it. In the patient's chart, we as nurses—and doctors, of course—have full access to all the patient's private information, including the medical history and corresponding diagnoses. The admitting diagnosis was for the stroke (CVA). But right after that, all other diagnoses were listed. The one listed right after the CVA was congestive heart failure (CHF). So the patient had been taking the loop diuretic Lasix.

Lasix was the first medication I ever administered to a patient back in nursing school. This medication's action takes place in the loop of Henle within the kidneys and is potassium (K) depleting. This medication is aptly named a "loop diuretic." This medication is utilized to reduce the body's fluid volume to reduce the risk of fluids backing up into the lungs when the heart isn't working sufficiently as a pump, and to decrease edema in general from fluid overload. The diagnosis, or its definition of CHF, is "the inability of the heart to work sufficiently as a pump."

The saline IV bag arrived to the floor in a one-liter bag with the 10 mg of potassium (K) mixed in. This, as well as the patient's name, was written right on the label, and all seemed in order. Darlene took the IV bag into Mrs. Kindle's room. Since Mrs. Kindle had a CVA, she was unable to verbalize her needs, so they had to be anticipated by the nurses. Darlene connected the tubing and fastened it to the patient's heparin lock, the IV port in the vein taped to Mrs. Kindle's left arm. With the bag hung and the port accessed, Darlene calculated the fluid-drop ratio on the IV infusing machine. The ratio of drops calculated would allow the entire saline bag's contents to infuse into Mrs. Kindle in one hour, per the doctor's order. Darlene pushed the start button, and the saline and potassium fluids began to drip. Darlene then left to attend to other patients in her charge, and I did as well with the patients under my charge, when all this was going on with Mrs. Kindle's medication flowing per doctor's orders (DO).

A red flag of caution obviously should be raised when putting anything into patients. A nurse should analyze the order, the history of the patient, and all the corresponding diagnoses and allergies.

I had worked for a nursing registry as well. I was staffed at one of the largest medical hospitals around on the ninth floor in Panorama City. I had an African American male patient with a diagnosis of sickle cell anemia, an illness that causes severe pain in the joints. The patient was complaining of this pain, and I looked in the MAR for the medication and the doctor-ordered strength. Demerol, 325 mg intramuscular (IM). The most I had ever given was 125 mg IM. Not taking the order as gospel, I checked it with the doctor's orders in the patient's chart, which read 325 mg IM. Still concerned, I asked the med-surg charge nurse.

She explained, "He's a frequent flyer here. He's been in and out with us for years. The order is correct. He has just built up a tolerance to the medication, so we titrate the amount up over time."

Only then did I draw up the Demerol and administer it.

I don't know what Darlene was thinking, truly an oversight of the CHF diagnosis.

With the continuing drops, Mrs. Kindle's heart pumped with increasing exertion. Like a clogged sink only allowing a remnant of the fluid to pass, it backed up. Blood flooded the chambers of her heart. Blood flowed back into her lungs via the pulmonary veins. I can't imagine the panic Mrs. Kindle felt, probably a feeling of being buried alive.

Darlene walked back into Mrs. Kindle's room an hour later to remove the empty saline bag only to find that Mrs. Kindle had drowned in her bed of an excess of body fluid. With the stroke (CVA) she was unable to move and unable to speak. With each drop of fluid came shorter and shorter breaths. It was a tragic oversight that killed Mrs. Kindle very slowly over an hour. This hit Darlene so hard that she was never seen again in any of the hospital halls. Termination was a sure bet for this reason.

28

Presidential Advice

Two days went by, and I was again working the long-term unit. I had just come out of a patient's room. Looking west down the hall to my left, I saw a man in a white shirt and tie, brown pleated slacks, and black shoes. He had short, receding brown hair, graying at the temples, and wore thick silver-rimmed glasses.

The man was the president of the hospital, Colin Weise.

He stopped five feet from the nurses' station, looking left and right while standing still in the middle of the hall.

Mr. Weise stated, "I need all nurses that had anything to do with the care of Mrs. Kindle to come with me."

He led us west down the hall and into an office. We filed in, and he pulled the door closed.

He stated, "Anyone who has no knowledge of this patient, leave now."

Two people left, one a certified nursing assistant and the other a nurse. He shut the door again and turned to face us five remaining nurses who knew what had happened.

Mr. Weise said, "If anybody comes in to ask questions about Mrs. Kindle, you are only to say, 'She…just…went…bad!'"

He held his hands two feet apart, waist high, palms down, and fingers spread open, and his arms rose and fell with each word.

She…just…went…bad. It echoed in my head.

I thought, *Now I'm part of a wrongful death cover-up.*

I stood void of feeling in my entire body, except for the taste in my mouth that was acrimonious. Mr. Weise nodded as if to get a chorus line of nodding heads in agreement with him, his eyes darting back and forth from one nurse to the next.

"OK then, thank you," Mr. Weise said.

He walked past us to the shut door, paused, and turned his head back to the left as if to add a closing thought. Saying nothing, he turned away, opened the door, and left.

I thought, *Maybe the look was a silent threat.*

We stood in silence staring at the open door.

"*So!*" I exclaimed. Everyone jumped.

"Don't, William," Riva said, despairingly soft, placing her hand out and brushing my arm in protest.

"I'm sorry. I just wanted to see if everyone feels like I do," I said.

I placed my palms flat on my white 501 jeans and wiped them dry from sweat.

I thought, *I don't recall ever having sweaty palms in the past.*

Problems were getting bigger, complicated, and the world was getting smaller. Smaller in the sense that the usual number of people you cross paths with on a daily basis, say hello to, or whatever may be increasing, shrinking our comfort in the world. And just yesterday I, for one, thought I had a handle on it—my world, that is. A woman is dead forever. If I didn't report it, "advocate" for the patient, I would be held just as accountable as the nurse who killed her. I was pretty sure this conversation from the president was the last part of the cleanup, as any paper work that remained was changed or destroyed. I had nothing to move forward on except word of mouth. Conspiracy, obstruction of justice—just saying it, I felt like I was drowning.

We all exited the office and went back to work. As I walked, I thought, *Should I be asked by a family member, or lawyer, a question regarding Mrs. Kindle, could I make them believe? Should I even try? With no way to prove it, would I be sued? Fired for sure.*

I tried over and over saying it in my head, practicing the lie, the deceit surrounding the death of another human being. A gun wasn't used, and I'm positive Darlene had in no way wished harm on Mrs. Kindle, but she was dead forever nonetheless. The family never to know the truth.

I thought, *She just went bad. Hell! With a liter of water in the lungs, who wouldn't?*

The thoughts continued. *What if I don't pull it off? What if someone else drops the ball, and I'm caught in a falsified cross fire?*

Serious, fearful pictures in my head of a distraught, grieving husband or daughter asking, "Why? What happened?" flowed through me. I saw myself in court on a stand, failing to defend myself. Criminal anxiety crept in, and sweat seeped through my palms, soaking my hands.

Every day I entered the hospital, I waited to be approached by Mr. Weise and told to accompany him again into a room of shirts, ties, and briefcases. After four days I began to settle back in the routine of work and normal breathing. I never was approached, and to my knowledge no one else was either. No one spoke of this tragedy.

I thought, *I wonder how this affected everyone else involved.*

How the others fared mentally, I'll never know; we never spoke of it.

It was about a week later that I was called into my director's office.

I first thought, *My worst fear for the month was about to come true.*

I was wrong; it was my second. The resource nursing director, Mandy, was a professional lady, almost fifty with dark hair with occasional strands of gray. She was well dressed and sincerely congenial.

She said, "I'm going to have to terminate you, William."

The way she said it gave me a feeling that someone else was pulling her strings. She was nervous.

Shocked, I asked the obvious. "Why?"

"Patient abandonment," she replied.

I asked, "Who, what, and where?"

Mandy continued, "I can't give names. That's confidential."

Mandy only told me it was from the long-term floor, like throwing me a hint.

The floor where I corrected the other nurses from overdosing Mrs. Colwell, about crushing the sustained-release 90 mg of morphine that was contraindicated. It was where I took the verbal lashing from Rachel, who gave me the scrub top for a gift. The same floor where I stepped in for Riva and explained about the catheter to Dr. Moore, for Mrs. Kindle.

The same floor where I was to keep my mouth shut about the wrongful death of Mrs. Kindle. I was tossed out like a used tissue after two years without a blemish. I would *never* abandon my patients.

A removal of loose ends is what this was. Throwing a few possible rats off to save the ship. This was a scare tactic. And it worked.

I was very concerned about the disciplinary action Sacramento was going to impose upon me with such a severe breech of professional etiquette such as abandonment. I thought, *How can I fight what I was sure to be me against two or more nurses who stated they, too, were crushing the medication that was overdosing Mrs. Colwell? Or Mr. Weise, implicating me in the wrongful death of Mrs. Kindle.*

Abandonment? What patient? I thought.

All questions and no answers. I waited for a suspension—or worse, a revocation in the mail of my nursing license—something that never came. This is because Mandy had assured me that "they," the hospital, weren't going to communicate it to the capital, another protocol not followed. And it never was communicated to the capital. The real reason was the fact I never abandoned anyone. They abandoned me.

29

A Traveling Break

With everything that happened in the halls of this hospital the past two years, I was in need of a vacation. Not necessarily from work, just from the drama of the hospital in general. Still maintaining my commercial driver's license, I hired on with a large trucking company out of Phoenix, Arizona.

I figured I would travel the United States and be paid for it. I was right.

It was mandatory for all new company drivers to undergo six weeks' training on the road. Supervised by another seasoned company driver, instructed in training new-driver hires.

Don Roe was my assigned driver. I made one attempt at humor about Don's name in reference to the Hawaiian singer Don Ho, and Don said, "I've heard 'um all." I let it go right there.

Don was a white male of thirty-three years of age with thinning dark hair and a black moustache. He was about five feet eight with an average build and had a great sense of humor. We spoke of past occupations, and Don told of his desire to become a fireman. We were driving west on I-40, between Flagstaff and Belmont, Arizona. Due west, we had the sun setting at just the right altitude in the sky to keep us company, face to face.

Don stated, "I had tried for seven years. All the hose pulling and non-paid brush clearing and so forth. I finally got my interview for a position with the fire department. I was friends with the chief and other higher-ups. They were all good guys, professional. At the beginning of my interview, I was sitting in an office, opposite five firemen. My chief turned on a tape recorder and stated my name, the date, and the reason for the interview. Then he shut the recorder off.

"The chief said, 'Don, we could spend the next hour going through the motions here, but I'll tell you right now, we hired someone else yesterday, an African American woman. My hands are tied.'"

Don remained silent after this statement and continued to drive west into the sunset. I looked over at him from the cab's passenger seat.

I said, "Well! Look at it this way, Don. If you had gotten hired at the fire department, I'd be getting trained right now by an African American woman."

I don't know if it was because we were tired at the end of a long day of traveling or because of my execution of my comment and timing, but we laughed generously for the last mile before shutting down for the night.

30

A Break on the Road

Years earlier, when I was eighteen, there was a radio station in our little valley of Simi. The call letters were KCME, and I was offered a DJ position there. One might say I had the gift of gab. And on many occasions, the owner, Rob, would run into the studio and wave his hands, palms down like he was pushing air toward the ground, mouthing in silence, "*Slow down*," so as not to be heard over the radio—wanting me to slow my speech down. With thousands of albums to play, I had full autonomy in what songs I played during a four-hour broadcast. I made innumerable amounts of tape recordings. Well edited. No commercials. I took these and many other self-made and professional tapes on the road. After a few days observing my driving, Don felt comfortable enough with my abilities to control the eighteen-wheeler, and he slept while I drove. We covered more miles. We were traveling east on US 80 in Wyoming. It was two in the morning and slightly snowing. I put on one of my favorite recording artists, Gordon Lightfoot.

I saw Mr. Lightfoot in concert at the Universal Amphitheater in Universal City, California, with my girlfriend Yessenia. She was from El Salvador and was twenty-three, ten years younger than me. Black hair waved in curls about her shoulders, and her black eyes were voracious. She had a figure that wanted for nothing. We were at the Universal City Walk, in Universal City, for dinner and noticed the marquee with Gordon Lightfoot's name. He was to perform that night. We immediately went to the ticket window and asked if there were any tickets left. We were told yes and shown a map of the amphitheater. Having worked a ticket-sales booth at a hometown record store called Tape King Stereo in Simi Valley, I was very familiar with the layout of the amphitheater. The map showed a small gathering of maybe ten rows of seats in the orchestra. Then the rows elevating up started with AA, followed by BB, and so on till EE. Then the loge started. The two available tickets were for seats BB, right on the aisle. I didn't hesitate. We purchased them. We walked in, and I bought a beer and Yessenia a glass of wine. We walked into the auditorium, vast and theatrical. The energy was exhilarating. We continued all the way down to the stage, two seats from the floor, two seats from the aisle. Sitting down, we had two big smiles. I had introduced Yessenia to Gordon Lightfoot's music a year earlier, and she was equally enthusiastic. About forty thousand fans filled the place. The lights on the stage came up in blues and reds with cuts of orange fading in and around the edges. The curtain came up and the sharp, clear, troubadour sound flooded out. The music and lyrics mesmerized. Mr. Lightfoot played for about two hours straight. He walked to the edge of the stage and spoke with the audience. He said his son and family were here tonight. He shook hands with people in the front orchestra seats.

He then said, "We're going to take a break and return in a half hour."

People jostled about, heading for restrooms and to the exits to smoke. After another beer and glass of wine, Yessenia and I returned to our seats, and Gordon Lightfoot returned to the stage. After another two hours of great music, the song I believe everyone was waiting for began with the foreboding, distant guitar's intro of an audible, impending doom: "The Wreck of the *Edmund Fitzgerald*."

It was a true story of a ship that sank in Lake Superior, taking all twenty-nine souls down with her—a poetic lament.

The amphitheater erupted in cheers, and everyone rose to their feet. I was right. Darkness came up, and everyone sat down in anticipation. After the song ended, people rose again. It was his last song, and he was shaking hands in front of the stage, moving from one side to the next. To the right and the left of the entrance to the stage were very large staff guards in yellow shirts, their arms crossed, spaced about ten feet apart. Everyone continued applauding. And as I did, I walked down the two steps that put me flush with the orchestra floor. I walked while clapping, smiling past the goliath sentries, their faces and bodies inert. Mr. Lightfoot walked to the back of the stage to exit through the red cloth curtains to his left. He remained waving to the exuberant fans. I walked up to the stage, which was about five feet high. I reached up over it and called, "Gordon!" loud enough that he looked back at me and came back out onstage, to the edge. I held my hand out, and Gordon shook it. I know by the look on his face, he wondered who I was, from my bold approach.

Gordon said, "Have a good night," still shaking my hand.

I said, "I already did, thank you!"

Having let go of his hand, I stepped back and clapped as he waved back to the crowd. Gordon walked back across the stage to the red draped curtain, waved, and then disappeared behind it. I went back to my seat where Yessenia stood slightly jumping up and down, elated.

She said, "You shook his hand!" while she took my right hand in both of hers. I laughed.

"Yes, yes, I did. Let's go," I said smiling.

We traversed up to the main-entrance floor and separated to adjacent restrooms. Standing in a long line, a young man in front of me turned and looked at me then turned back.

He turned again and said, "So you got to shake Gordon's hand."

I paused. I looked around at the masses of people ambulating in all directions. I looked back at the guy and replied, "You recognized me from all these people?"

He said, "Yes. You were on the big screens. Wherever Gordon Lightfoot went, the cameras went. You were shaking hands on the big screens that give a view to people sitting farther back."

I replied, "I didn't think of that. We sat two steps up from orchestra. The screens were well behind me."

"Nice seats," he said.

"Yeah," I replied, a thousand-yard stare on my face.

I was thinking I could sneak a handshake off to the right of the stage, and no one would know but me and Mr. Gordon Lightfoot. I was wrong.

As Yessenia and I buckled in for the drive back to Simi Valley, she asked, "What if those big guards caught you?"

I replied, "Then they would have probably kicked us out. But it was the end of the concert, and had they, we would be the first ones out of the parking lot, and first still on the 405 freeway. No traffic!" I smiled and filed out of the lot.

No traffic at two in the morning on US 80. The truck rolled east between Laramie and Cheyenne, Wyoming. Snow flipped about the windshield, a skein of white butterflies in appearance, magnified by the headlights and darkness of the interior of the cab, which resembled a Winnebago motor home. The only interior lights came from the amber instrument panel from the dash. Don slept in the sleeper about four feet behind me. My Gordon Lightfoot tape played, and one song faded, and another started. A perfect setting, traveling down a lonely strip of blacktop in the middle of nowhere. Darkness to the right and the left. The only thing that gave me a sense of earth's chronological time line was the rig in which we rode. All else was millions of years old. The next song started with an unmistakable, ominous moan: "The Wreck of the *Edmund Fitzgerald*."

The song played like a movie soundtrack over the scene, and tonight I could have been on my own perilous journey. I could have been in the wheelhouse of the ill-fated *Edmund Fitzgerald*. As the song faded away, silence filled the cab. I felt empathy for the crew of the *Edmund Fitzgerald* and their families.

"William!" Don said in the silence, interrupting my thoughts.

"Yes, Don. Too loud?" I replied, referring to the music.

I turned my head toward the back of the cab and sleeper compartment, where Don leaned up on his left elbow.

Don said, "No, not at all. In the past week, I've heard songs I haven't listened to in twenty years and new ones I love, and I haven't heard one twice. You have impeccable taste in music, William."

I replied, "Thanks, Don. The musicians make the music. I just put them in the machine."

Don got up and came to the front of the cab; sat in the passenger seat; and lit a smoke, cracking his window to vent the smoke. Cold, brisk Wyoming winter air blew in from the dark night.

He said, "Pull off in the next turnout, and I'll take over."

"OK," I replied.

Don looked down at the radio. "Who was the artist of that last song?" he asked.

I picked up the cassette case. "Gordon Lightfoot," I said, and handed it to him.

"Mind if I listen to it?"

"Not at all. Help yourself to any of them. No worries."

A few miles later, we came upon a turnout, a black, paved notch area off the road. The only other thing in the turnout was a trash can encased in a chain-link fencing to keep the bears and other wildlife out.

I pulled in, stopped, and set the breaks. Getting out, we stretched our legs. Snow was five inches deep on the ground opposite the road on both sides. White, unblemished sheets reflected an ice-blue tint from a now-clear, starlit night.

Staring up, I thought, *The night is as black as sackcloth that may have been used to catch a porcupine. The millions of holes left from quills allowed brilliant light through, like the sun was placed just behind it.* It was a view rarely seen in the smog-cloaked skies of Los Angeles.

The only thing remotely close to a cloud was the white fog from our breath against the black, sackcloth night. Don and I walked around the rig and trailer. Checking lights, kicking tires, we performed a general inspection, and then we mounted back up in to the cab. Don shifted up ten gears and then popped the cassette into the player. I lay down in the back bunk to listen to "The Wreck of the *Edmund Fitzgerald*" and five encores before Don let the tape play all the way through the rest of the tape's selections, ending with one more repetition. It was readily apparent that Don more than just liked the song. It was a great combination of journey, night, weather, geography, topography, and song that made for an unforgettable memory of the road.

We drove together for about two weeks, from Oxnard, California, to places like New Jersey; Memphis; Amarillo, Texas; and small towns I'd never heard of. I admired the roadside mom-and-pop cafés. Rest areas set in ancient forests.

The Painted Desert of New Mexico. Then we drove west again, returning to Don's home in Twenty Nine Palms, California. We drove in on a back road, worn, uneven, and infested with potholes, through an open desert of mesquite bushes and wind. Sporadic homes sat in the dust. Slowly we rolled past a couple of houses and pulled to a stop on a dirt road. In front of the last house, the dirt road continued and dissolved and was reclaimed back into the desert a quarter-mile out—an ironic, fitting end to our travels.

Don pulled the air brakes, and swirls of dust blew out from both sides of the rig with an exhausting hiss. He turned off the ignition, and the tractor shuddered as the diesel engine stopped. Don sat up straight, peering out across the desert landscape.

He said, "You know, you don't have to stay the last four weeks. You were good to go after the first one."

I nodded my head, said nothing, opened the door, and got out. After a stretch, I unloaded my bag. I pulled two full plastic grocery bags of tapes out. I fished out the Gordon Lightfoot tape. I packed up my car, which had sat in two weeks of desert dust that turned my black Toyota Camry tan.

I thought, *At least the word "Love" that had been scratched on my trunk in the hospital parking lot is covered.*

With the thousands of miles I just traveled, the hospital felt far away.

I started my car and let it idle. Don came out of his front door to see me off.

"You good?" Don asked.

"Yes, I'm off to Simi."

"I'll call Phoenix and tell them you need your own rig. It'll be out of Ontario, California."

I said, "Thanks for your time and company, Don. I really enjoyed it."

"It was my pleasure. You're the best trainee I've ever had."

I pulled the tape of Gordon Lightfoot out of my back pocket and handed it to Don. "Some traveling tunes for you," I said.

Don accepted it, shook my hand, and thanked me.

I said, entering my car, "See you around the beautiful rest areas that divide the ruins, Don!" I put my car in drive and headed south for the 10 freeway.

31

Treading Not So Lightly

had put off driving for a few months and worked for the nursing registry that staffed major medical facilities in and around San Fernando Valley, California. I figured the winter months would be over, and I could start fresh come spring. And being a nurse, or in any profession really, requires one to remain sharp—can't be away for long periods of time.

Summer rolled around, and I reported to Ontario, California, to a large company terminal. I was assigned a one-year-old clean white Freightliner and received a load and headed out to Phoenix, Arizona. I was hired to drive the eleven western states. After dropping my trailer in Phoenix, I got a message on my onboard computer, called a "Qualcomm." It gave my next destination. I was to take another trailer to Georgia. Atlanta, to be exact. It was, however, my prerogative to take the run or not. I did. My whole reason for taking time off from the hospitals was to relax and explore the road and other states and towns. I hooked up my assigned load, a fifty-three-foot trailer, and exited the terminal. I turned onto the 10 freeway and headed out east again toward Georgia. When I made Louisiana a couple of days later, the sky was dark from rain clouds. It rained so hard, big rigs and cars alike had to pull to the shoulder. It was as if a fire hose had been turned on full and aimed at the windshield. Over the CB radio, I asked, "Is there a truck stop close by?"

A man's voice came on and stated, "There's only a minimart off the next exit; that's all there is for miles." I thanked him with a double-click of the handset. There was a chord of static and then silence in the cab.

Outside, the rain beat down like falling marbles on the roof. I spent the night parked in the market's lot. So did six other rigs. I slept and waited the storm out. The next morning, I awoke to a host of orange warmth. Steam rose from the rain-soaked blacktop. I continued east down the 10 freeway. The drive went uneventfully till halfway through the state of Louisiana where I drove past a tire tread that had come off an eighteen-wheeler. It sat on its edge, a black three-foot strip of rubber, seven or more inches high, its length across the middle of the fast lane. Using my side mirror, I watched an approaching car. Behind it was another car that, for the speed it was doing—about seventy—should have been farther back. The first car bore down right up to the tire tread.

I thought, *Don't do this*, observing from my rig's large side mirror.

I could see a white male behind the wheel. His intentions were clear as well as highly reckless. Just at the last minute, he swerved right from the tread into the only other eastbound lane. The car behind him reacted accordingly and swerved hard right, even harder than the front car due to reflex and surprise. Overcorrecting to the left, toward the middle divider, the brown midsize car flipped sideways and rolled. The first roll launched the car in the air; it came down and continued for another three. The divider was very wide and full of browning summer grass, three feet tall. Dust and twisted debris flew up in a cloud of devastation. The vehicle came to rest upside down, something I had witnessed firsthand while driving an ambulance. I pulled my truck off to the shoulder and set my breaks and emergency flashers. I got out, locked the door, and jogged across the two-lane highway and into the three-foot thicket of the divider. Two men squatted down by the driver-side window. I wore blue jeans and a white T-shirt; black work boots; and a black cowboy hat I bought at a truck stop at midnight in a blizzard outside Laramie, Wyoming, seven months earlier.

I pulled it off my head and said, "Hi, guys, I'm a nurse and a paramedic. Can I be of help?"

My words barely finished, and the two men stood up and walked away in opposite directions. I stood alone, grass up to my thigh and an upside down car to my left. In my personal vehicle, I carry a ditty bag, a nick-name used by medics for a collection of medical supplies. But I wasn't in my car. Placing my black hat on the bottom of the car—now the top—I knelt down and looked in the broken driver-side window. I observed a white female—about forty-five years old with black hair and a medium height and build—lying on her back on the inside roof of the car, which rested in the same position in the weeds.

No seat belt, I thought.

Her eyes were open. Her face pale and in shock.

I said, "Hello, miss. My name is William. I'm going to help you. Everything's going to be fine. I won't leave you. And I'm a nurse."

Recalling what I looked like, I smiled and said, "I know I don't look like it."

This was my second day without shaving, and my hair was pulled in a shoulder-length ponytail.

"Will you tell me your name?" I asked, calmly assessing the broad picture of the smashed interior.

"Linda," she answered in a shallow voice, almost a whisper.

I was a bit relieved. By the contorted shape of the steering wheel above her head, it was possible she had sustained a chest injury, possibly with broken ribs and punctured lungs. I kept speaking to her.

"Where are you coming from, Linda?" I said, wanting to keep her talking, as to assess respirations and level of consciousness.

Linda replied, "From work. I have lab specimens in my trunk." She spoke clearly and concisely.

Labs? I thought. This raised a red flag of caution.

I asked, "Are the labs something we should be concerned about?"

"No" was all she said. I kept the labs on a shelf in the back of my mind. With my commercial license, I had the hazardous-materials endorsement. Any spill or contaminate had to be communicated.

I continued my assessment. No cyanosis (blue) about her lips, and her face color had returned to a pale rose. No blood on the anterior, or front, of her chest, and symmetrical chest expansion might rule out a pneumothorax, or sucking chest wound, that would allow for one or two of the lungs to collapse if punctured. On Linda's left arm, right at the elbow, was an avulsion—a chunk of flesh torn out, leaving a gaping hole—that was bleeding slowly. I expected profuse bleeding from such a wound. However, it could have been worse if the injury breached her brachial artery, under her humorous bone above the elbow.

I palpated Linda's extremities. I asked, "Can you feel this?" and squeezed Linda's left foot.

"Yes," she replied.

"And here?" I squeezed the other foot.

"Yes."

No broken bones. No further bleeding besides the left arm. Linda remained dazed but alert and verbalized appropriately. Other cars had stopped as well. I looked back and saw several people standing about. I recalled, when I used to drive the ambulance, the slowing traffic on the 101 freeway in Los Angeles years prior, with onlookers of similar situations. It always angered me.

The temperature now was one hundred degrees with humidity at 90 percent. Sweat ran down my face. I kept swabbing it with my shoulders. My T-shirt was already soaked through. Looking out at the people from my crouched position, I made eye contact with some and looked across the rest.

Might as well use them! I thought.

I raised my right hand high in the air to get their attention.

I exclaimed, "There's a lot of people here!" My voice rose louder. "And I'm sure it's because you want to help!" The crowd stared back at me.

I continued. "I need bottled water, unused, the cooler the better. And any first-aid kits you might have. And I need them now!" People moved in all directions, heading for their respective cars then coming back over to me with all I asked for.

Crossing that ever-elusive path of compassion for another again. I thought, while wiping another sweat drop, or tear, from my eye.

One car had just pulled to a stop, and a young white female of maybe twenty-five got out wearing hospital scrubs. She was blonde, cute, and athletic. She grabbed a bag from her trunk and quickly joined me. Kneeling to my left, she placed the bag on the ground, opened it, and pulled out two sets of surgical gloves.

Handing me a pair, she said, "My name's Monique. I'm a nurse." She looked down at Linda and then back up at me. Her blue eyes increased the Louisiana day's heat.

I replied, "A ditty bag. Thank you, Monique. My name is William."

We donned our gloves as I spoke. "Monique, this is Linda."

"Hello, Linda," she said, and gave a compassionate smile.

I said, "Linda is alert and oriented times three. Pupils PERRL"—pupils equal, round, reactive to light—"steady pulse of eighty. Respirations twenty and unlabored. Other than being a bit shook up, the only obvious injury is a small cut here on her left arm, as you can see."

I looked at Monique. She looked at the avulsion and back at me and nodded. I was impressed by her professionalism. She knew my comment about a simple cut was made not to distress Linda, still lying inert on her back. Monique assisted me as I asked for supplies. I leaned inside the car and over Linda. Opening a new bottle of water, I irrigated the wound. I took sterile four-by-four gauzes from Monique. I wet them and cleaned the dirt, glass, and blood from the left arm and the avulsion. I looked around the glass and other debris for the missing part of Linda's arm, hoping to save the chunk of tissue, but I found nothing to put on ice.

Monique soaked large gauze pads and put them around Linda's neck and to her sides. Cooling measures from the heat. Three police cars finally rolled up. Four police officers in all got out.

I thought, *We must be a ways off the beaten track here.*

It seemed to take a while for a response. One officer approached us and stood by the rear of Linda's upside down sedan. I asked the officer for the estimated time of arrival (ETA) of the ambulance, and he told me it was called when they were and should be arriving any minute. Monique and I advised the officers that we were nurses. The other cops began to disperse the crowd and directed the congested traffic. I packed Linda's arm with a wet-to-dry dressing of the sterile four-by-fours and wrapped it with a roll of four-inch gauze. I smelled the vapors of gasoline and looked out and to my right. The gas-tank-filler cap was on this side of the car, and fuel was leaking and running down its side. The heat, the dry brown grass, the fuel—all the ingredients to make a bad situation worse. I couldn't move Linda for fear she might have a spinal injury. But burning would surely expedite the demise of everyone in the immediate vicinity. I tapped my fingers on the side of the car while looking up at the police officer still standing by. He looked at me and then at the car as I pointed to the spilling fuel, and then he looked at me again and nodded. He quickly went to a police cruiser and got a fire extinguisher and stood vigilant at our side. I could hear some of the officers telling people to keep moving.

"Who's in the big rig over here?" an officer asked loudly.

I pulled my head out of the window and raised my right hand.

"That'd be me, sir!" I said while my right hand extended high up. My gloves were bloody. A small piece of serosanguinous—or bloody—tissue flipped off my glove behind us and fell to the ground.

The officer immediately said, "Never mind. You keep doing what you're doing." I nodded and turned my attention back to Linda.

The ambulance finally arrived. It pulled past us and parked. It was on the opposite side of the wreck. A large dark-haired man exited the unit. Short and blunt, heavyset, weighing about 270 pounds, he meandered in our direction. Tracking around the back of the car, he bent down to see his reflection in the rear passenger-side window, which was still intact and tinted. He calmly adjusted the dark, plastic-framed sunglasses on his face. Looking at him, I then turned my head and looked at Monique, who shrugged, equally as confused as I was.

"Stay with Linda, Monique," I stated.

"I'm here," she replied.

I got up and walked a few steps from the car and past the ambulance driver who stood idly by. Then I ran across the weeds and tall grass to the ambulance that sat with the rear doors farthest from the crash. The norm would have been to pull the doors closest to the patient, making readily available all medical supplies within. I rounded the back and opened the doors. Sweat stung my eyes, and I brushed them with one shoulder, then the next. A man of maybe seventy-five sat looking through the unit's cabinets.

Another brief moment of disbelief on my part.

I said, "I need the gurney, a full-length backboard, a cervical collar, two small sandbags, and a roll of tape!"

The man turned and looked back toward the cabinet.

"You might find the tape in there," I said, and entered the back of the unit.

I pulled the backboard out of a wooden slot and laid it on the gurney. Opening a plastic see-through glass slider, I pulled the C-collar and threw it on top of the backboard. A roll of white dressing tape hung from a silver-tipped oxygen port protruding from the unit's wall. I pulled it off and stuck it in my back pocket.

I asked the man, "Can I get you to step over here?" and motioned toward the front. He stood and complied. I opened the bench seat he'd been sitting on and retrieved two small sandbags. Closing the bench seat, I thought, *Ambulance supply storage hasn't changed a bit.*

I placed the bags next to the C-collar and jumped out the back of the ambulance. I reached for the latch that released the gurney and pulled. Rolling it out, I released the wheels connected to the steel rails, and they unfolded and fell to the ground. I made the gurney level, standing four feet high, and then I lifted and dragged it through the weeds and waffled dirt from city tractors that cut the divider's grass (but not lately, I assumed). Monique was still kneeling down by the window and Linda. The police officer with the fire extinguisher stood by the fuel tank while the other three continued traffic control. The ambulance driver remained standing idle in the weeds. Undoing the gurney's belts, I took the cervical collar and knelt back into the broken window.

I explained to Linda, "I'm going to slip this collar under and around your neck. It may feel uncomfortable, but it's necessary to keep your head and neck straight, OK?"

Linda said, "Yes."

Monique and I then rolled Linda's body in unison and slipped the backboard under her, placing the two sandbags on each side of her head.

I pulled the roll of white dressing tape from my back pocket and ran three long strips over Linda's forehead and fastened the ends under both sides of the backboard. Two officers and Monique helped me lift Linda to the gurney and strapped her securely with the safety belts, immobilizing her. Full C-spine precautions. I remembered the dips in the dirt and didn't want Linda jostled across the field.

I said, "I need a man on all four corners of the stretcher."

Two police officers took a corner, and the ambulance driver and I took the other two. We lowered the gurney to the ground and the wheels locked in place. Lifting, we walked to the rear of the ambulance and locked the gurney in place. I advised the driver to drive out over the divider slowly, which he did.

Back at Linda's mangled car, Monique was standing with her medical bag over her shoulder.

She said, smiling, "I don't know what you're doing driving a truck. You missed your calling."

I replied, "I've heard that said. But driving a rig takes skill, too. I'll return to the hospitals in time. Right now, though, I'm on vacation." I laughed.

Three of the four officers offered handshakes. I accepted.

One officer said, "She was lucky you were here."

I replied, "Thank you, sir."

Monique gave me a hug, turned, and walked back to her car.

Retrieving my hat, I walked back across the grassy divider. Grasshoppers were jumping everywhere. I hadn't noticed them before. I stopped and looked back at the brown sedan lying on its roof in the grass. Looking down, I brushed some of Linda's sedan's chassis dirt off the rim of my black cowboy hat and put it on my head. I turned, and when the road was clear of traffic, I crossed the two-lane 10 highway back to my rig.

After reaching Atlanta, Georgia, I picked up pesticides going back across the entire country to Fresno, California. Important paper work was involved with this hazardous material. It gave off a strong, pungent smell of chemicals. The pesticides were locked in several sealed containers. And there were a couple of restrictions on where I could and couldn't drive. I knew whatever driver was used for this load, the driver had to have a hazardous-material endorsement. That was a given. I remembered what Monique said, "What are you doing driving a truck?"

I thought, *Don't ever underestimate the importance of someone's profession.* The trip went smoothly. I didn't glow in the dark after, either.

32

The Roads Commencement

I could feel the road had run its course after almost a year. I was ending my last runs before returning home for good, to another hospital, and to Yessenia. Heading to the first of my last-three stops, I drove east from Seattle, Washington. It was getting late, and my drop had to be before seven.

I missed my drop outside Moses Lake, Washington. It was eight o'clock and dark. I shut down for the night at Ernie's Truck Stop, off the 90. I backed my truck in between multiple rigs idling in the dirt lot. Windows were covered with silver windshield blinds. I often wondered where they all drove in from and where they all were going. The road can seem timeless. The next morning early, I climbed down from the rig and walked across the dirt parking lot. A gray fog had rolled in during the night and hovered above the ground. I entered Ernie's Truck Stop. Bright florescent lights constricted my pupils as they adjusted. The smell of fresh coffee led my way. My coffee in hand, I paid and walked toward the door.

"Have a good day, and drive safe," the clerk said with genuine sincerity.

I turned and looked back to the counter. "And to you. Good day and thank you," I replied.

The dawn crested and revealed a canvas of lavender to the east. The fog dissipated, leaving only a faint mist that lay in the low parts of the fields that surrounded the truck stop. Stars faded to the west. From my cab, I drank my coffee. I rolled out and made my destination and dropped my cargo.

The onboard computer directed me to proceed to Lewiston, Idaho.

Off the 90, southeast of Moses Lake, Washington, I drove down Route 21.

On all sides of my truck, I could see nothing but fields of gold wheat. I pulled over on a very small strip of dirt, parked, and shut my engine off. I climbed down from the cab and walked west from the truck and into the field. Wheat as high as my hips, it grew from horizon to horizon. The silence was such it made my ears ring, except for a crow on occasion in the distance. I stood still and gazing at as close to forever as I'd ever come.

I thought, *How lucky we are.*

A breeze moved the tops of wheat in swaths. The sun was warm and heavy, hypnotic, giving me a feeling of sedation. I pulled off a handful of kernels. Looking around, I thought; *Time to go home—back to Simi Valley and back to Yessenia.*

I walked back toward my rig, which sat motionless and silent across the gold abyss, while chewing on my stolen blessings.

Many miles, many roads. Many beautiful rest areas that divided the ruins. And I never did cross paths again with my driver trainer, Don Roe.

33

Part of the Tribe

Yessenia and I had moved in together after the six months that I had been out on the road. I had made it home every two to three weeks approximately, and now we lived in a two-bedroom apartment in Simi Valley's east end. I wasn't home a week and was already working at the nursing registry that staffed medical facilities in and around San Fernando Valley. I was scheduled at a hospital in Panorama, a med-surg floor I had been on in the past. Receiving a paper that would be filled out by the charge nurse for the floor, an evaluation, I took the elevator up nine floors and onto the unit. There were five nurses on this unit with six patients each. The patient report was given, and we went to work. Something about registry personnel—we always seemed to get a condescending, cold-shoulder welcome, like we were outsiders, not part of the tribe. This was true this evening. Another nurse came in—Vicky, Filipino, about forty, short, and heavyset. About every hour, she needed to ask me if I had done a treatment or given a medication. After the second hour, her routine had run its course.

I said, "We work out of the same books here. If I signed it, I did it! If I didn't sign, I didn't do it," We stood face to face at the counter that supported the two books I pointed at.

She replied, "Well, we need to keep checking registry nurses. They miss so much."

"And what have I missed?" It was a rhetorical statement. I turned away and entered a patient's room. My patient was a white male, thirty years old. He weighed six hundred pounds but was on a strict diet now and fluid restrictions. He kept asking for water, and I kept explaining why I had to deny him. He was incontinent, so it was necessary for the other four nurses to assist. It's a precarious thing to roll someone this size on his side, four feet from the floor. Everyone helped roll and hold while a CNA cleaned him—everyone but Vicky. Two other Filipinas and a white nurse were always accommodating. I started IVs and such for them, if and when they asked. One of Vicky's patients was an elderly white male. He was confused, so soft ties were applied to both wrists to quell his combativeness. He had a triple-lumen catheter in his right carotid artery and an indwelling urinary catheter. Vicky had found more time to shadow me. Her malevolent behavior was obvious to everyone working the unit. Going about my duties, both mentally and physically, I noticed an abrupt change in the other four nurses as well as the charge nurse for the floor. From the elderly man's room, they came in and out double time.

I walked over to the front counter to check a doctor's order in one of my patient's charts when I was asked from across the room, "William! Do you have a tourniquet?"

Looking toward the voice, I saw three nurses, all with their hands in an IV kit box the size that would hold one pair of shoes.

I patted my pocket and calmly said, "No, I don't have a tourniquet."

I lifted one of the floor stethoscopes from a doorknob. These floor stethoscopes were made of hard, plastic tubing.

I said, "Bring the IV kit," as I was now aware that it was Vicky's elderly patient they all had their attention on. I walked into the patient's room, where I observed blood sprayed about the walls. The confused elderly patient had escaped one hand from his restraints and pulled the triple-lumen catheter from his right carotid artery. Blood sprayed from his neck. The bed, floor, and walls looked like some horror-movie set. On the floor lay the patient's urinary indwelling catheter; the 30 cc balloon that keeps it in place within the bladder was still filled. The norm would be to aspirate the 30 cc of saline before removing the catheter through the urethra. Pulling the blood-soaked sheet away, I observed that the patient had himself pulled this catheter out as well, and the pressure of the saline-filled balloon split his penis in two like a banana peel. I knew these nurses were determined to get an IV started as soon as possible because of the amount of blood loss. I still had no tourniquet, so I wrapped the stethoscope I brought from the doorknob around the patient's left arm and pulled it moderately tight.

The patient's basilic vein protruded, and I said, "Stick him."

An IV was inserted with little effort and the bag of saline hung. I completely opened the roller that controls the amount of fluid to infuse (the acronym TKO means "to keep an IV open completely") We placed sterile four-by-four gauzes on his neck, with one nurse holding pressure. Another nurse had called the doctor, and soon he was being rolled out of the unit for surgery toward the elevators and out of my life. I never saw him again; how he fared I'll never know. Now it was clear, having basically orchestrated this emergency, that I was on everybody's good side, including Vicky's.

Feeling like a captive, though, now I was made one of the tribe.

34

Patients' Advocate

I walked into the long-term-care facility I had resigned from a year before (to once again drive eighteen-wheelers around the country) with two boxes of doughnuts, one for the front station, and one for the back. A woman I did not recognize greeted me, and I introduced myself and told her I was a former nurse employed here before venturing out on the road for a year. She was the director of nursing. Her name was Raja.

So I was back in the setting of this long-term hospital, or more technically described as a "convalescent hospital," a misleading term meaning recovery. Misleading especially for an individual of ninety years old, give or take a year or three.

I met all the characters of the play that was to unfold. Or maybe it'd be best described as an opera, a more despairing scene of events that portray the evils of selfishness.

The director of nursing, or DON, was Raja Homes. She had the corporate attire and the condescending air to keep the peasantry at bay. She'd arrive in the morning about nine and take a brisk walk around the facility floor, which was a perfect square. A good morning here and there and then the inevitable, "I have a luncheon meeting," and then she was gone for the rest of the day, breaching the facility's door only one other time in the late afternoon to clock out.

She was a brunette woman around forty years old, slim with a handsome physical appearance. My obvious disdain for this woman was not immediate.

The director of staff development, or DSD, was Liza East, RN, a thin, plain-looking woman of thirty-something. Her hair was medium length and dirty dishwater in color, and she was about five feet five. She'd held a couple of in-service meetings about the expectations of employees, all ranks. We sat through the videos of recognizing patient abuse and the protocol in reporting it, as well as the repercussions of not reporting such a professional breach of etiquette.

The videos, I had seen before, as they shared universal knowledge in all hospital settings, especially the video on sexual harassment. It is my opinion that these lean more toward the male stereotype: the sleazy, balding, middle-aged man groping his secretary. And why not? Any attempts at portraying a dominant woman in an offending sexual situation fell easily into the category of embarrassing, at least in these mandatory videos we were subjected to.

After Liza, the DSD, pushed the start and stop buttons of the machine playing out these videos of banality, we were all excused back to our floors and stations, or home, if the mandatory in-service fell on your day off.

Then Liza would walk about the halls that divided the patients' rooms and go out the southeast door to the back of the facility to smoke.

That's if she didn't accompany the DON, Raja, on one of the mandatory luncheons every day of the week.

Roberta Rhine, LVN, was the floor charge nurse, the same position and title I fell under. We had an even number of patients divided between us. She, like myself, would dispense medications and monitor four to six CNAs. She had blond hair with no real style other than it was there, pulled up in failed attempts at correcting the obvious. She was about five feet seven, 145 pounds. Again, my disdain for any of the individuals staffed at this hospital was not immediate.

Roberta had been a licensed vocational nurse for ten months. At this time I had been licensed for ten years and had worked many of the surrounding facilities, so I had met and treated more than a few of the patients that resided at this long-term-care hospital in my hometown of Simi Valley.

I knew of my patients' diagnoses and with them their individual limitations, from fluid restrictions and allergies to foods and, just as important, medications. With all patients, regardless of the setting, came their living wills, which stated their desire to have, in case of a life-threatening situation, either efforts taken to revive them or a do-not-resuscitate order (DNR).

Within a week of working at this facility, and already very familiar with the day-to-day routines, I was to cover two night shifts because of a call-off. With the eleven-to-seven shift came some minor changes in responsibilities. One of these was to change the 60 cc syringes utilized to access the gastric-tube sites of patients who could not consume food, water, or medications by mouth (PO).

At midnight all 60 cc syringes were collected, and new sterile ones would be dated and have the patient names and bed numbers written on the outer container that held the new sterile syringe within. And during my regular day shift, the other day nurse and I would be the first to breach the sterile seals when performing the morning medication pass. Most days I worked with Roberta Rhine. Some days with another nurse and the occasional change of sides of the hospital.

This was a good way to keep knowledge of all the patients within the facility and maintain a higher level of care. Some patients were admitted for CVAs or strokes, and most were admitted due to the passage of time and the gradual limitations that inevitably came with it. They needed assistance with their ADLs, or activities of daily living: dressing, eating, walking, and personal hygiene.

With some diagnoses, like a stroke, the ability to verbalize one's needs were severally limited, if not all together lost. One of a nurse's skills in a situation as serious as this is to anticipate the needs of the person. Observation is equally important for all patients, of course.

Here is where the question comes in from my assistant director, Mrs. White, ten years prior, during my nursing-admission interview: "What do I mean by being the patient's advocate?"

About the second week, as I walked down the hall, I observed a female patient who I'd known well for the past three to four years and had treated in another facility unaffiliated with this one before being transferred here.

We'll call her "Lady." Lady was approximately forty years old. Your first thought might be that that is such a young age for anyone to be a resident in a long-term-care facility. Lady had a diagnosis of "neurological unspecified."

There was something wrong with Lady mentally that was "unspecified" because even though she had been through many tests, doctors were unable to find and cure the ailment that caused her loss of speech and range of motion (ROM) and left her with no other way to communicate than to cry. Any person being bedridden for years will atrophy, a medical term that means to deteriorate, wither, waste away.

Lady's only means of mobility was with the assistance of certified nursing assistants; physical therapists; and, of course, us nurses to reposition her for comfort and ADLs. My emphasis on this condition is in hopes that not only medical professionals but we as human beings should never lose sight of how lucky we are with our health, as well as how tragic someone in Lady's condition is. And those who choose a career in health care should never lose sight that they are this "patient's advocate."

I approached Lady, who lay in her bed that had been brought into the hallway. Her hands and feet contracted from muscle and tendons distorting and pulling her extremities inward, painfully inward. Tears ran down her face, and she grimaced in obvious pain.

I greeted Lady and said, "Why are you hurting so terribly?"

Of course all Lady could do was stare up at me, right into my eyes. Anyone could have heard her cry for help through her eyes.

Where's Lady's nurse? Her advocate? Where's Roberta? I strained in thought.

I worked this side of the floor on occasion and knew that Lady was to be given routine pain medications. These were medications with exact times to be administered. Confused, I walked down the hall to advise

Roberta Rhine, LVN, of, on this day, her patient's condition. Roberta was nowhere to be found. I asked Roberta's sister, who worked supply, where I could find Roberta, and I was told she didn't know.

I walked to the medication cart for all the patients on that floor. I turned to Lady's MAR, which listed all medications and times that were doctor ordered to be given, and all medications had been signed by Roberta, meaning that all medications ordered had been given. Using the key to the lock of the cart, I opened it and checked all medication packets for the date and medication for that morning. All medications were gone for their specific date and times.

The morning medication pass for approximately thirty-eight patients took at least two hours. I would go toward my patients' floor, and Roberta would go to hers. Each of us had our own medication carts; each of us had the same amount of patients in our charge. Again, I'd been licensed for ten years, and Roberta ten months.

Out of curiosity I kept an alert eye on Roberta's routine and found that it took me two hours to complete my morning medication pass, but it took Roberta only fifteen minutes. After completing our medication pass for that time, both carts would be put back in their place just outside the nurses' station.

So after we had started, I noticed Roberta pushed her medication cart back in place fifteen minutes after rolling it down the hall to administer her patients' medications. I feel it necessary to place emphasis on that these patients are our family members. Perhaps not by blood, but definitely by human association.

I watched Roberta then walk down my floor toward the back of the hospital. At this end was the kitchen, maintenance room, and the south exit where those who smoked would go out to the designated area for that purpose. Roberta entered the maintenance room. I then walked around to check on Lady and a male patient who was admitted for a stroke.

A stroke, as I've explained at times in this book, left one paralyzed on one side of the body, depending on which hemisphere of the brain was affected.

Also, stroke could cause loss of speech. Few had the ability to verbalize their needs, and even then it came in very slow, slurred, and almost always unintelligible attempts.

And there was the frustration that went with this communicational handicap.

With the stroke came the inability to swallow in most cases. And with this inability came the necessity of a gastric-tube insertion. With this tube the patient was fed, medicated, and given water. To be sure, all stroke patients would have one specific medication routinely given, often referred to as an anticoagulant. One commonly used was called Coumadin. This medication was a blood thinner. It was utilized to decrease the risk of another stroke from occurring and, in some cases, help expedite recovery.

We'll call this gentleman Walt. His room was right next to Lady's. As I walked past his room, I observed him sitting in his wheelchair beside his bed. He was more in a slouched position as his ability to reposition himself due to the paralysis was very limited, if it existed at all. His curtains were closed, and there was no light on, and his room did not possess a television set. It was almost noon, and the room was as dark and gloomy as if it was past eight at night on a cloudy day. Next to him was a machine utilized to administer a liquid diet, his only source of nourishment. Depending on the doctor's order of how much each individual patient was to receive, these machines could run 24-7. Walt's wasn't running at all, and the tube that would connect to his gastric tube (GT) just hung down the length of the machine; a few drops from the residual feeding fluid had dropped to the floor and coagulated in a puddle.

From having worked this floor on many occasions and my knowledge of these patients, including Walt, I knew his feeding tube should not only have been connected but running as well. I took Walt's 60 cc syringe off his bedside table and twisted the cap off, at which point I felt the sterile seal break. This was very much a surprise to me as the seal should have already been breached from the first time it was used to administer his morning medications.

I removed the unused 60 cc syringe from its casing and accessed Walt's GT. Customarily, the syringe tip is inserted into the gastric tube, then I would pull back on the plunger of the syringe to aspirate, which would show how much, if any, residual fluid remained in the patient's stomach. Walt's held none. I then aspirated 30 cc of water from his bedside water pitcher and flushed his gastric tube. This is done to clear the tube of any possible occlusions, like feeding solutions that had set up within the tube and clogged it. I then started the feeding machine, or IVAC, and allowed the fluid remaining in the tube to run out into a cup till the length of the tube's contents had run out and fresh fluid began. Attaching the feeding tube to the GT, I pushed the start button, and his nutrition infused.

I opened his curtain and his window half a foot for ventilation and sunlight. I assisted Walt in sitting up straighter in his wheelchair and employed a couple of his pillows to help keep him braced comfortably. I wet a washcloth and wiped up the puddle on his floor. Exiting his room, I threw the cup containing the feeding solution in the trash.

One door down I entered Lady's room and found her in the same condition as before: rigid and in tears. I immediately took her 60 cc container from her bedside table and found it, too, had not been used. I did the same for Lady as I did for Walt and then left her room. I went directly to the nurses' station, and once again Roberta was nowhere to be found. I opened her MAR and found all meds were again signed for, and upon viewing the medication cards, I saw that the medications were gone.

A question of an obvious nature came to mind: how can you give the medications and increment of water via a gastric tube without first removing the syringe from its sterile sealed container?

The only answer was, "You can't."

And where was Roberta? Where was these people's advocate?

On the next day, after the morning medication pass, I went to Liza, the director of staff development. I would have gone directly to the director of nursing, Raja, but she was out again on another "luncheon."

I asked Liza to accompany me into both Walt's and Lady's rooms. I showed her my concerns, which were extremely obvious.

Liza, looking down at the unused 60 cc syringe, replied, "This is her second time."

I then said, "Rank and file."

Liza replied, "What's that?"

I explained, "Now the ball's in your court. As the director of the development of this facility's staff, I have brought a concern of patient abuse to you, per policy. This was on the video you showed the newly hired, myself included."

Liza nodded yes in agreement.

I recalled lying awake at night, wondering about all Roberta's patients. "Did they get their meds? Their water?"

Well, now I knew this concern, red flag, this *criminal neglect*, would be rectified.

The next day Roberta and her sister were speaking at the nurses' station.

Roberta's sister Rose, who was about three hundred pounds and always spoke louder than necessary, said, "Who told?"

Roberta replied, "William. Liza took me out back for a smoke and told me."

I was going about my duties and glanced at both of them.

A day had passed. I was sitting at the nurses' station, doing paper work of one kind or another, when I overheard Roberta's sister announcing to a CNA that Roberta was once again pregnant. I was unaware that she had any children.

"How does Juan feel about it?" Roberta's sister asked.

"He's fine. We already have one, so what's one more?," Roberta replied.

So it became clear what it was Roberta spent her time in the maintenance room doing with Juan the maintenance man while her patients lingered in dark rooms with no medications; no food or water; and no advocate, save me.

I'd have thought that since Liza and I were both aware of Roberta's neglect, she would have taken better care of her patients, her responsibilities. But it didn't change a thing. She continued her mornings as if nothing happened. It was so blatant, I felt like I was being tested to see if I'd approach this red flag as dictated via the videos on this very situation.

35

Sexual Request

The following Saturday, Liza walked down the hall toward the back nurses' station where Tina (the RN) and I sat doing paper work. Tina had what was routinely Roberta's side of the hospital, and I was maintaining my usual side.

Liza was dressed casually. Her face was devoid of expression. "I need to talk with you right now!" Liza said, pointing at me with her arm extended almost all the way.

Tina turned her head toward me and rolled her eyes like she was saying, "What's this about?"

I shrugged and stood up, pushed my chair in, and exited the station toward Liza.

Just as I approached Liza, she turned and started to walk up the hall, away from the nurses' station. Just when I thought she was going to stop and turn to talk out of earshot of Tina, Liza again turned and proceeded up the hall and around the corner. I followed her and soon came to the director's office door at the front of the hospital. Inside was another nurse working on material-data sheets on a computer.

"Connie," Liza said.

Connie turned and looked at us.

"Yes, Liza?" Connie replied.

"Can you excuse us for a moment? I need the office," Liza said.

Connie looked back at the computer screen and back toward us. With a two-handed knee slap, Connie implied that she was doing her job, and Liza was causing her an inconvenience. Then Connie walked out the door, and Liza motioned for me to enter first. It was about noon, and I was a little inconvenienced myself. I had to check blood sugars on my diabetic patients and give them their routine insulin as well as any regular (R) insulin in accordance to whatever their blood-sugar levels were. And it needed to be done before the patients ate lunch, which was just then being pushed down the hallways in stainless-steel meal carts by dietary workers.

Liza pushed the office door closed and turned the dead-bolt lock. I stood facing her about seven feet away.

"What's up, Liza?" I asked.

I was thinking it definitely had something to do with Roberta and the patient neglect on her part.

"My husband lives in a vodka bottle. I've been sleeping on the couch for the past eight months, and I want to fuck you," Liza stated verbatim.

It's been a practice of mine not to make decisions, or in this case, a reply, on emotion. I stood motionless and in thought. Not a thought of how to respond, but more of, *Did I hear that right?*

It was surreal to say the least. Then I thought, *The audacity.*

I chewed on this while contemplating a window of escape.

To swallow would be to answer, so I just said, "This is going to make for a lousy work environment." I was thinking out loud for sure. I needed out of this situation, yes, but first I'd take getting out of this office, and Liza stood between me and the only door to the outside, which just then someone knocked on. At this time Liza had stepped up to me and stood like a sixteen-year-old prom date waiting for her kiss good-night.

"I need to get back to work!" Connie's voice exclaimed from the other side of the door where safety lived.

I'm usually in control in stressful situations, but this one left me feeling trapped. Connie knocked again.

OK, time to expedite my departure, I thought.

"Liza, I have a girlfriend, and you just said you have a husband. I just moved into an apartment with my girlfriend of three years," I stated while pressing around one of three desks in the office, the desk corner sharp against my thigh as I moved toward the door, where Connie knocked again.

"Hello!" Connie repeated.

"I know you just moved into a new apartment, and that's why I'll pay for any hotel or motel, but I can't have you driving past my house!" Liza said, clearly delusional, in a world of her own.

"This isn't going to happen, Liza, so damn-small chance of that happening," I replied, somewhat sternly, as I was getting angry at how presumptuous she was.

I thought, *How do I get out of this, and what am I looking at in terms of retaliation?* With my experience in the past, there was always retaliation.

One thing at a time, I thought, but Liza still prevented my escape. I didn't want to touch her even to move her to the side. This could get very ugly. Should she become angry at my failure to reciprocate her desired objective, she might say that *I* was the harasser. And who would believe me, a man? This was as tough a spot I could ever remember being in.

I thought, *It would be far easier bronzing an ice sculpture.*

The next knock came as if a US Marine wished to enter.

Knock, knock, knock!

This seemed to jar Liza into some degree of normalcy, at which point I placed my hands on top of her shoulders and guided her away from the door.

Looking at her this close now, Liza's eyelids were heavy, and she appeared to be sedated to a degree, lethargic. I smelled no alcohol, but at this moment I knew for sure, and not just because I'm a nurse, Liza was under the influence of something of a controlled substance.

I reached and turned the lock. Opening the door, I could see that Connie was upset. I just exited and walked the distance to the back nurses' station, stepped past Tina, pulled my chair out, and sat down. I could feel Tina looking at me.

"What happened?" Tina asked.

"It wasn't a talk she wanted," I replied, never looking up from the patient chart that lay on the counter in front of me.

Nothing came up of a retaliatory nature after this particular event, in no way, shape, or form. And I was surprised, agreeably.

36

Director's Disregard

Days later the director of nursing (DON), Raja, had stayed within the hospital. Again, the patients left in their state of neglect, I walked into the DON's office where Raja sat speaking to the administrator, Kate.

Kate was nice enough and greeted me accordingly when I entered the office.

"Raja, can I speak to you?" I asked.

"Of course, William," she replied as she stood and walked toward the door where I stood.

"I'd like to share something with you," I said, and motioned with my hand in the direction of Lady's and Walt's rooms a few doors down the hall.

"I'd like to see if you can pick out what's wrong with this picture," I said, standing at Lady's bedside.

Raja looked at Lady, the bed, and Lady's meager possessions.

"Look at the 60 cc syringe, please," I asked.

Picking up the syringe encased within its see-through plastic container, Raja looked it over and glanced at me.

"Open it," I said.

Raja placed her hand on the top and attempted to slide off its cover, which should have been with ease. When the cover refused to slide off, Raja grabbed the top and with modest effort twisted it, and the top came off with a snap sound that came with the sterility seal being broken.

Raja slipped the syringe out and looked up at me. It being twelve o'clock in the afternoon, Raja knew this particular syringe would have already been utilized a few times. She also knew the seal had just broken.

Raja asked, "How is she getting her meds?"

"Raja, she's not!" I replied. "Didn't Liza tell you of this issue?"

"Well, she may have mentioned something," Raja replied, still looking blankly at the dry syringe and its container. When used, there would be condensation in the container as well as the syringe itself.

Reiterating the whole story, I advised Raja of Walt, and most certainly all of Roberta's patients, of the time in which Roberta performed her morning medication pass, or rather of the time she didn't.

I told her all about Roberta, Juan, and their expanding family.

Raja nodded her head and walked out of Lady's room and into Walt's to find the same results. Raja then walked to the MAR, the med book that rested on top of Roberta's medication cart. She turned to Lady's med sheet and looked at all the morning medication times that again had been signed.

"May I use your keys, William?" Raja asked.

"Of course," I replied, handing them to her.

Raja opened the medication cart and looked at the medication cards that came with each medication in a bubble with corresponding dates; there was no doubt that many concerns were warranted.

Raja locked the cart and handed me my keys.

"Thank you, William," she said as she turned away with determination.

I felt relieved and disappointed. Relieved that I wouldn't be spending anymore nights lying in bed, staring at the ceiling, gnawing over what had not been done for Roberta's patients, and disappointed that Roberta, or anyone, could be so uncaring toward another person, especially under these circumstances.

I knew hospitals didn't hold the monopoly on neglect of any kind, or degree.

I had a thought about my next plane flight somewhere, and did the person responsible for tightening the bolts that held the wings on take as little care with the bolts as Roberta did with the patients in her charge?

The next day I had off, but there was a mandatory in-service with a doctor, a personal friend of mine. The in-service was of a pulmonary nature. After the in-service ended, I walked out the front door where my car was parked.

As I shut the door and placed the key in the ignition, an abrupt elbow came in through my driver-side window, which I had rolled down.

"Ay, man! Chu betta start havin' respect for Roberta!"

Startled, I had turned and was face to face with Juan, the maintenance man of this hospital, and Roberta's baby daddy, as I knew they weren't married. His Mexican accent was thick and intimidating.

Before I knew it, I was out of my car and standing inches from Juan.

"Respect for that?" I retorted, while pointing enthusiastically toward the facility.

I don't remember opening my car door, or even touching the door handle. I handled this street situation verbosely.

"Fuck you! And her! You haven't a clue what's going on here!"

Now as I advanced on Juan, he stepped back with his hands up shoulder height as I flagrantly explained my world he had entered uninvited.

His facial expression was now one of surprise and confusion.

"You're right, man! I don't know what's going on," Juan volunteered in his slow, but steady retreat.

I turned back toward my car, now half a parking lot away, but kept my head turned enough to see Juan for the first five steps. As my car door was already open, I got in, pulled it shut, and left.

Who are these people? Where'd they come from? This was truly amazing. Amazingly terrible. Could it get any worse? I thought.

37

Sick Termination

The eighth week back at this facility, with all this manifesting, I came down with an upper respiratory infection (URI). Just before four in the morning, I called, per hospital policy, and true of this one, as a cold for me might mean pneumonia for the patients, especially in a geriatric setting. That was known as a "nosocomial infection," an infection you bring to work with you.

I called and spoke with Dale, the night RN I was supposed to relieve in the morning. Also per policy, if you're not able to make your scheduled shift to work, a two-hour minimum notice must be given.

I dialed, it rang twice, and the phone picked up.

"Hello, nurses' station. This is Dale."

"Good morning, Dale, this is William," I said.

"What's up?" Dale asked.

"I won't be in today—something's really got me sick."

"You sound like shit," Dale said.

"Yeah, productive cough, fever," I replied.

"OK, I'll communicate it to Raja when she gets here in the morning."

"Thanks, Dale."

"No problem, Will," Dale said, and hung up.

I stayed at home and with a tympanic (ear) thermometer monitored my temperature that was now 102. I was shaking from feeling cold still. I was wearing three shirts and a flannel.

At eight o'clock I called to speak with Raja, the DON. I was told she wasn't in her office. I left a message for Raja with the receptionist. Raja never returned my call. Since I'd only been back to this hospital just less than two months, my medical benefits wouldn't go into effect for another month, but my concern for my illness was increasing along with my temp, now 103.

About ten I called back, and Raja took the call.

"Raja, I'm really sick, so much that I want you to know I won't make it into work tomorrow either. My temp is 103.0," I explained.

"That's OK, William, you're terminated anyway!" Raja stated in a matter-of-fact tone.

"Terminated! For what?" I exclaimed.

"No call, no show," Raja replied.

"I called. I spoke with Dale. He'll corroborate my story."

Anything was a possibility with this bunch. *Was this retaliation? But the sex thing, that was Liza, not Raja,* I was thinking.

"Well, I'm coming in, Raja! Right now," I said.

Living close to the facility, I was there in five minutes and rolled into a parking spot, got out, and entered the hospital. I walked into Raja's office, where she sat behind her desk.

"This is bullshit, Raja! I called in three hours before my shift. I called in!" I exclaimed.

I realized I had my arms crossed the whole time, as I was still cold. I placed my right arm between the back and seat of one of the swivel chairs, picked it up, and threw it at the wall that divided the administrator's office and Raja's. Kate, the administrator, was in Raja's office within seconds. I continued to reiterate all I'd had to contend with the last eight weeks, and, yes, I used some strongly worded references.

Damn it! Who the fuck do they think they are? Don't they know this is somebody's living they're playing with? To use and toss out like a used tissue, I thought.

Kate, about sixty years old with white hair, stood just inside the office door. She was looking at me as I took a chair. I was winded, and my wheezing could be heard without the use of a stethoscope.

"You know, William, you really don't look well," Kate said.

"And I feel worse than I look," I replied.

"Maybe you should go home and rest," Kate said.

"No, first I want Liza brought in here. I'm going to tell you something else that happened no less than a week ago, right here in this office!" I exclaimed.

A passing CNA was delegated to locate and deliver the message to Liza.

"I got Roberta throwing the patients' medications away, neglecting them in every way, and I bring it to your attention. I got Juan accosting me in the parking lot! And when Liza gets in here, I'm going to tell you what happened, and Liza's going to do one of two things. Get angry and deny, or try and rationalize it," I said with my arms crossed, and rocking slowly back in forth in the chair.

Just then Liza entered the office with a look of confusion mixed with a touch of fear.

"A week ago you brought me in here 'cause you said you needed to talk to me, dismissed Connie from this office, and then shut and locked the door. Then you turned to me and stated, 'My husband lives in a vodka bottle, and I've been sleeping on the couch the past eight months, and I want to fuck you.'"

Liza stood inert, in shock.

"Well…I, um…" was Liza's reply.

"Liza! I want you to leave the office right now!" Raja exclaimed.

Liza didn't hesitate.

"William, you should go home now and rest," Kate urged again.

"You're not getting it. I'm suing all of you! And before I die," I retorted. "I'm so fucking tired of taking this shit. Everywhere I go, it's like I've got a sign on my back saying, 'Fuck me over.' I'm not going home; I'm going to Dr. Corbin, chief doctor of this facility. I'm going to have him diagnose me so I can document my illness for court. Dale will be called, Dr. Corbin, and, of course, you!" I yelled at Raja, throwing my hand in her direction.

"What will be your defense, Raja, when asked what did you do for those patients who were being neglected? Why wasn't Roberta reported for elder abuse, if not criminal abuse? And lest we forget the ever-articulate Liza! I think we all know how she'll fare under questioning."

I got up and advanced toward the door. Kate stepped to the side, giving me a wide berth.

"I'm suing all of you," I stated once more as I exited the office.

I drove the two blocks down to Dr. Corbin's office and went in. I've known Dr. Corbin for years, having worked other hospitals in Simi, Thousand Oaks, and the San Fernando Valley.

Dr. Corbin was speaking with one of his receptionists as I approached the front desk.

"William, what…you look…" His words didn't finish.

"Come back here." Dr. Corbin directed me as he opened the access door to the exam rooms.

"Have a seat," he said as he applied his stethoscope. "Deep breath," he said, moving the stethoscope over all five lobes of my lungs, anterior and posterior.

I began to once again have one of my coughing episodes and grabbed a tissue to hold over my mouth. Upon stopping, I expelled the contents of my productive cough in the tissue, a thick, green sputum. Dr. Corbin placed a thermometer under my tongue. He then pulled a prescription pad from his white lab coat and sat at a seat with a small ledge protruding from the wall. Dr. Corbin finished writing and tore the page from the pad and left it on the counter. He pulled the thermometer from my mouth.

"It's 104.1," Dr. Corbin stated as he looked directly at me, his concern obvious. "You're going to get a blood draw. I want a complete blood count (CBC). And you're going to need a note for work. I'm going to admit you into the acute hospital for IV antibiotics," he said.

"No, thank you, Doctor. I won't need a note for work; they terminated me a half hour ago. I called in sick, but Raja said I was a no call, no show and fired me," I explained.

"You have pneumonia, William! And I'm admitting you to the hospital now," he said sternly.

"I've only been back eight weeks and don't have the six hundred dollars a day to lie in a hospital bed having some nurse do for me what I can do for myself at home," I stated.

"Go get this blood drawn. I want it stat!" Dr. Corbin said.

I left and went to the lab in the acute hospital, where a vial of blood was taken. I then returned to Dr. Corbin's office, where I went back in the exam room and lay on the examination table. Dr. Corbin had called the lab, and the results of my blood work returned via a fax. Dr. Corbin walked just inside the exam-room door, and I sat up. He handed me my lab sheet and walked out. Usually, it's the nurse calling the doctors with abnormalities found on a patient's lab sheet. I had sent these kinds of sheets or called Dr. Corbin many times regarding them, so when he handed it to me, I knew that *he* knew that I'd understand what I was reading. An elevation of white blood cells (WBC) is indicative of an infection. A normal level is between 4.0 and 11.0; mine was 15.0.

"You need to go in for IV antibiotics," Dr. Corbin advised again.

"I can't afford that right now," I replied.

"I will admit you, and I will write the whole thing off!" he stated.

A gleam of hope filled me. Hope for mankind. I found myself crossing that rarely crossed path of compassion.

"I tell you what! I'll give you antibiotics by mouth now, and you have two days to improve, or I will admit you and write the whole thing off!" he repeated. "What the hell is going on over there?" Dr. Corbin asked me.

I reiterated the story. "Do you want to know why your Dilantin levels or Coumadin levels resemble an EKG strip, Dr. Corbin?" I referred to that strip of lines that spike up and down with the rhythm of a heart. I continued. "Because when a real nurse works that floor, the patients get their medication. When Roberta Rhine, LVN, works it, she throws all the medications away and goes back to the maintenance room to fuck. That's why you've got peaks and troughs. That's why you can't get a therapeutic blood level," I stated.

I became winded again, so Dr. Corbin had me lie down for a while. After five minutes I took the prescription to the pharmacy and then took my sick unemployed ass home.

The next day, my temp was down, but still at 101.0. I couldn't relax—I was so angry. I had great concerns about the treatment of the patients left at that hospital. I called Ombudsman, a state group that advocates for patient rights.

I then booted my home computer and wrote a clear summary of the whole event. Two days later I drove out to Ventura. I went to the Department of Fair Housing and Employment. In a waiting room with more than thirty people, I waited my turn to speak about the injustice done. Not to me—although I was in the story briefly—rather I was there to focus on the needs of the patients I advocated for and my concerns about them. As I sat opposite the government employee who sat reading my story, he stopped and looked up at me.

"If half of what I've read is true—" he said.

Interrupting him, I said, "All of it's true."

He then got up and walked to his door and leaned out. "I have one here. I'll be busy with this one," he explained to someone I didn't see farther down the corridor.

Documents were given to me with their corresponding reference numbers, and I went home.

I realized that all my past employment references would be detrimental in getting another position. I had visions of walking into another facility with my résumé, to once again utilize a nursing license I worked very hard in obtaining. But knowing my past employers and experiences, my advocating for those who were ill, weak, and scared and some dying—the reason I choose to continue this profession would more than likely have to rely on others I have known, to see them and their families through such trying times. That's if you can find them.

38

Hearsay

One DON at a facility in the San Fernando Valley I interviewed with listened while I briefly explained my last position.

"I know all about it. I know your name and who you are. We have a third of that hospital's patients in this facility," she stated. "Orientation is three days long. You start tomorrow morning, eight o'clock."

I was happy I got the position and reported the next morning at seven forty-five.

During this first day of orientation, five other people, one other nurse, and I sat through those familiar videos of elder abuse and sexual harassment. Then we were taken on a tour of the facility—fire doors and extinguishers, escape routes and nurses' stations. The gentleman directing the tour then had us go outside to view the location of the emergency generator. Should there be an earthquake, or any other reason the facility should lose power, we had to know how to turn on the emergency generator to keep the machines powered—machines that keep ventilators running that patients rely on to breathe for them. Our small group of new employees meandered back down to the conference room when, out of the corner of my eye, I saw Tina, the RN from the other facility. Tina, with whom I had occasionally worked. Tina, who asked me what Liza wanted.

She walked out of a small office, holding some files in her hand. We made eye contact, and she walked up to me.

"I know you" was all she said.

She turned and walked toward the administration offices.

Whatever Tina said, her version of what was relayed to her by Raja, Liza, and Roberta was enough to send my resume into the nearest trash receptacle.

Shortly after I returned home from my first day of orientation, my cell phone rang.

"William? Hi, this is Kelly, director of nursing at—"

"Yes, of course, Kelly. What can I do for you?" I said.

"Well, I'm sorry, but I'm going to have to retract our offer for your nursing position," she said.

"May I ask why?" I asked.

"Yes, well, I had two women out on maternity leave, and they're both coming back, so I don't have an opening at this time," Kelly explained.

I asked, "So they both waited nine months to communicate this to you?"

"They weren't sure," Kelly said.

"OK, my best to you; the facility; oh, and Tina, of course," I said, and hung up, knowing I had again just been lied to. I felt some consolation in that it was a polite lie—no heroin solicitation; I didn't reek of vodka; and no depraved sexual comments to the female staff, patients, or farm animals.

Damn! Doesn't anyone have the balls to tell the truth?

It would be ten years before I got another nursing position in another hospital. My name was, and still is, well-known. My story—the version depends on who tells it—is equally known. So I continued with home health on occasion to keep up with my nursing skills.

39

"What Do I Mean?"

"What do I mean by being the patients' advocate?"

The question is as fresh in my mind as the day Mrs. White asked it.

"A voice for those who literally don't have one" was my reply.

Would I do it again? Would I speak out about neglect perpetrated by one of my peers? Yes! Yes, I would, as if he or she were doing it to me.

Ernest Hemingway wrote, "Man was not designed for defeat," and "The world breaks everyone, and afterward, some remain strong in the broken places."

Granted, he was a mortal man, and his writings weren't divinely inspired gospels. I just happen to agree with him, from my own experiences.

I have achieved much. I have lost much. I have contributed, and I have taken. I have been humbled, and I have been brave. With all the dark corners in my time, I have maintained courage enough to keep going in life and not give up—a resilience in self-preservation. I truly believe that I am one that has "remained strong in the broken places." A firm confidence backed only by the fact I'm still here.

www.ingramcontent.com/pod-product-compliance
Lightning Source LLC
Chambersburg PA
CBHW051912170526
45168CB00001B/344